Human B Cell Populations

Chemical Immunology

Vol. 67

Series Editors

Luciano Adorini, Milan
Ken-ichi Arai, Tokyo
Claudia Berek, Berlin
J. Donald Capra, Dallas, Tex.
Anne-Marie Schmitt-Verhulst, Marseille
Byron H. Waksman, New York, N.Y.

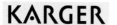

Basel · Freiburg · Paris · London · New York ·
New Delhi · Bangkok · Singapore · Tokyo · Sydney

Human B Cell Populations

Volume Editors   *Manlio Ferrarini,* Genoa
                        Federico Caligaris-Cappio, Turin

21 figures, 1 in color, and 5 tables, 1997

KARGER   Basel · Freiburg · Paris · London · New York ·
New Delhi · Bangkok · Singapore · Tokyo · Sydney

....

Chemical Immunology

Formerly published as 'Progress in Allergy'
Founded 1939 by Paul Kallòs

RC
583
.P7
v.67

Drug Dosage. The authors and the publisher have exerted every effort to ensure that drug selection and dosage set forth in this text are in accord with current recommendations and practice at the time of publication. However, in view of ongoing research, changes in government regulations, and the constant flow of information relating to drug therapy and drug reactions, the reader is urged to check the package insert for each drug for any change in indications and dosage and for added warnings and precautions. This is particularly important when the recommended agent is a new and/or infrequently employed drug.

© Copyright 1997 by S. Karger AG, P.O. Box, CH–4009 Basel (Switzerland)
Printed in Switzerland on acid-free paper by Thür AG Offsetdruck, Pratteln
ISBN 3–8055–6460–0

....

Contents

---

58 Subepithelial B Cells of the Human Tonsil

M. Dono, S. Zupo, C.E. Grossi, Genoa; *N. Chiorazzi,* Manhasset, N.Y.;
M. Ferrarini, Genoa

70 Malignant Lymphomas Stem from Different B Cell Populations

P.M. Kluin, J.Han, J.M. van Krieken, Leiden

85 What Do Chronic B Cell Malignancies Teach Us about B Cell Subsets?

O. Pritsch, K. Maloum, C. Magnac, F. Davi, J.L. Binet, H. Merle-Béral, G. Dighiero,
Paris

Preface

The idea of editing a book reporting the experience of several research groups on human B cell populations was conceived during the European Science Foundation (ESF) Conference on B Cells in Normal and Disease State: The Molecular Basis of Human B Cell Disorders, held in Lunteren, The Netherlands, October 14–19, 1995, and was fostered by Don Capra, editor of this series. At the Lunteren meeting, which gathered a fair number of experts on human B cells, it became clear that, along with the 'classic' topics of B cell investigations, such as the mechanisms of generation of antibody diversity and the early stages of B cell differentiation, a new research field was emerging, centered on the definition of mature subsets of B cells.

Until recently, the general understanding was that mature B cells were a rather homogeneous population of cells, the functions of which were simply to produce antibodies of increasing affinity and to maintain an immunological memory by transforming into resting, yet more easily stimulatable, cells. In this scenario, there was relatively little space for the concept that diverse B cell families could exist with different homing properties, surface markers and even specialization in the type(s) of antibodies produced. In addition, the complexity of the anatomical structure of peripheral B cell areas was not so well understood as to suggest ideas devoted to the existence of sites specialized in fostering peripheral diversification of mature B cells.

The possibility of fractionating peripheral B cells of humans and experimental animals according to the expression of the surface marker CD5 provided the first hint indicating the diversification of B cells. Compared to 'classic' CD5– B cells, CD5+ B cells produced polyspecific (natural) antibodies, had less stringent requirements for accessory cell support in order to be stimulated and apparently were characterized by different life span, homing and self-renewal properties.

A major breakthrough in the same field was the identification of the germinal center (GC) of the lymphoid follicle as the site where antigen-stimulated B cells complete their maturation process and are selected for their capacity to produce antibodies of increasing affinity. B cells exiting the GC either transform into antibody secreting plasma cells or enter the memory B cell pool. Studies with large panels of monoclonal antibodies have demonstrated that GC B cells, follicular mantle B cells, memory B cells and plasma cells can be phenotypically identified and purified in vitro. More recently, again using panels of monoclonal antibodies with B cell specificity, it was determined that the B cells of the splenic marginal zone, of the subcapsular area of lymph nodes, of the dome region of Peyer's patches and of the subepithelial areas of tonsils all share phenotypic and functional features which are distinct from those of the other B cell subsets.

While a large body of evidence was provided by studies on normal B cell fractionation, substantial information also came from observations on lymphoproliferative disorders. For example, most of the phenotypic and molecular properties of GC cells were determined by studies on follicular center lymphomas and also on Burkitt's lymphomas. Likewise, several of the unique features of the splenic marginal zone B cells and of their equivalent cells from other tissues were determined by studies on MALT lymphomas, that unequivocally derive from these cells. A contribution to the understanding of human B cell subsets also came from studies on congenital immunodeficiency patients. Both hemopathologists and pediatricians have taken good advantage of the new information, as documented by the fact that classifications of lymphoproliferations and immunodeficiencies are now largely based upon the new schemes of B cell maturation and diversification. Paradoxically, the emerging information has contributed to the casting of doubt on the 'traditional' CD5+ and CD5– B cell subdivision and the original classification (B1a, B1b and B2 cells) that was derived from this subdivision. Since CD5+ B cells appear to represent a subset of follicular mantle cells, at least in humans, the issue clearly deserves further debate.

Review articles by groups deeply involved in research on human B cell populations are collected in this book. Studies on both normal and malignant B cells are reported and in one article, the most important advances in the field of immunodeficiency are illustrated. These articles are preceded by a chapter on the molecular mechanisms underlying T–B cell interactions during the immune response. This information is necessary for the further understanding of the interactions that occur during a normal B cell response (or are faulty in particular pathological conditions). Although, it has been rather difficult to assemble the whole book, we have been rewarded by both the kindness and advice of our colleagues and friends and also by the interest generated by reading of all of the different opinions and speculations. Certainly, this is a field for active and most likely rewarding future work. We hope that the readers will prove to have the same interest we have had during our editorial work.

Manlio Ferrarini
Division of Clinical Immunology, Istituto Nazionale per la Ricerca sul Cancro, Genova
Department of Experimental and Clinical Oncology, Università di Genova, Genova, Italy

Federico Caligaris-Cappio
Cattedra di Immunologia Clinica, Department of Biomedical Sciences and
Human Oncology, Università di Torino, Torino, Italy

Contents

Ferrarini M, Caligaris-Cappio F (eds): Human B Cell Populations.
Chem Immunol. Basel, Karger, 1997, vol 67, pp 1–13

....

Molecular Mechanisms Involved in T-B Interactions

Peter Lane

Basel Institute for Immunology, Basel, Switzerland

The ability to generate somatic mutants and select them with high efficiency forms the basis of the capacity of mice and men to generate high affinity antibodies. The power of somatic mutation is enormous. From its repertoire of 200 million B cells, a mouse generates primary unmutated antibodies of micromolar affinity, comparable to artificial man-made immunoglobulin libraries of a similar size [1]. After somatic mutation and selection, the affinity of mouse antibodies is typically nanomolar, and to achieve this with man-made libraries without mutation would require a library size 10,000-fold greater [2]. This gives some idea of the benefits somatic mutation and selection confer on mammals.

Requirements for T Cell Priming

The architecture and cellular interactions which occur during the evolution of T-cell-dependent antibody responses are now fairly well understood. However, our understanding of the molecular interactions which guide lymphocytes is still rudimentary and there are many controversial questions. T-dependent antibody responses require cooperation between primed T cells and antigen-specific B cells along with effective help from accessory antigen-presenting cells. It is becoming increasingly clear that these different cell types are dependent upon each other for costimulatory signals which ensure that they differentiate and proliferate appropriately. This review will concentrate on the key decision processes which allow effective T-dependent antibody responses to develop, and the molecular interactions both known and speculated to play a role in this process.

Effective T Cell Priming Requires Reciprocal Costimulation between T Cells and Dendritic Cells that Involves Signaling through CD40

Under normal circumstances, initial antigen-specific T cell proliferation is associated with dendritic cells in the T cell areas of secondary lymphoid organs. Dendritic cells activate T cells potently, by virtue of their antigen processing capabilities [3] but also because they express costimulatory molecules such as B7 family members, high levels of MHC, and adhesion molecules. Dendritic cells also express and are stimulated through CD40, to become excellent APCs [4], expressing increased amounts of costimulatory molecules and producing large amounts of IL-12. T cell priming is poor in CD40 ligand-deficient mice probably because dendritic cells fail to get activated through CD40 [5]. This is not due to absence of B cell costimulation, as B cells are not required for normal T cell priming [6]. The mutual dependence on cells for their effective activation and differentiation forms a logical basis for maintaining individual microenvironmental niches within secondary lymphoid organs.

Role of Costimulation through CD28 and CTLA4 in the Regulation of T Cell Clone Size

The presence of costimulatory molecules of the B7 family on dendritic cells means that they can effectively signal T cells through CD28 and on activated T cells CTLA4 [7]. Most attention has focused on costimulation through CD28 [8] but it is now clear that signaling through CTLA4 negatively regulates T cell responses [9, 10].

The role of CD28 in T cell priming is controversial. There is no doubt that costimulation through this molecule amplifies T cell responses, but T cell priming occurs in animals in which costimulation through CD28 is blocked, suggesting that it is not absolutely required [11, 12]. What is not in doubt is that effector immune functions dependent on T cell help are severely compromised in mice where CD28 signaling is deficient, showing that CD28 plays a key role making CD4+ cells help antibody and cytotoxic T cell responses [13, 14].

Negative Regulation of T Cell Clones

Overemphasis on the idea that absence of costimulation is responsible for the induction of anergy has distracted attention from the alternative possibility that T cell clones are actively controlled by negative regulation. Two molecular mechanisms appear to play an important role in this process. The first is Fas and its ligand; mice deficient in signaling through this pathway develop autoimmune disease in susceptible strains of mice, and accumulate T cells [15]. The normal deletion which follows T clonal expression after immunization does not occur [16].

The second and apparently distinct mechanism involves CTLA4. CTLA4-deficient mice die early from a lymphoproliferative disorder [9, 10]. Fas ligand-mediated killing is preserved, suggesting that these two molecular mechanisms work at least partially independently of each other and are not redundant mechanisms to control T cell clone size. This could be explained if they operated in independent microenvironments, failure in either mechanism independently leading to disease. For example Fas ligand does not seem to play a role in the regulation of germinal centers [17], and one possibility is that clonal expansion of germinal center Th2 cells is exclusively regulated by signaling through CTLA4.

Whereas the triggering of Fas ligand leads to cell death, CTLA4 signaling leads to prliferative unresponsiveness (anergy) [18]. CTLA4-expressing T cells are found in the outer T zone and within germinal centers [19]. Recently it has been shown that at least one mechanism of action of CTLA4 is to recruit a phosphatase to the TCR, downregulating signaling [20]. CTLA4 may play a crucial role in regulating T cells not accessible to fas ligand, as is probably the case within germinal centers. The threshold for inducing T cell proliferation is much greater than that required to elicit T cell help. In this respect both CD28 and CTLA4 may act like a thermostat on signaling through the TCR, initially amplifying CTLA4-negative CD28-positive antigen-specific T cells, and then downregulating CTLA4 expressing activated T cells to a point where they are effective helpers in the selection process of germinal center B cells, but do not themselves proliferate in an uncontrolled way. In contrast, Fas ligand exerts its effect by regulating proliferation in the T zones [21].

A Mixture of Th1- and Th2-Primed T Cells in the T Zone Ensures that B Cell Responses Here Are Carefully Regulated

In Fas ligand-deficient mice, there is exaggerated B cell proliferation and differentiation to antibody-producing cells in the T zones of secondary lymphoid organs [21]. While this might be due to exaggerated T cell priming, taken together with the fact that Th1 cells inhibit B cell responses [22], this argues that Fas ligand expressed by Th1-primed T cells plays a role in limiting B cell proliferation. Secondly, Fas ligand has been demonstrated to play a role in eliminating autoreactive B cells [23]. This control step works at the stage that B cells differentiate into effector cells, producing potentially damaging autoantibodies. Immune responses to foreign pathogens often elicit autoantibodies during infection and this may be an important mechanism to ensure that such responses are self-limiting.

What Determines Whether T Cells Effectively Help B Cells to Form Germinal Centers?

Some B and T cells activated in the T zone migrate to B cell follicles where they proliferate in concert [24]. This early clonal expansion is crucial to the subsequent events which allow efficient selection of B cells, as it ensures there are enough T cells to select postmutation germinal center B centrocytes. However, in mature germinal centers, most T cells do not proliferate, despite antigen-specific signals from B cells. As suggested previously, signaling through CTLA4 on these activated T cells may be responsible for this [20].

CD4+ cells can effectively differentiate into at least two types [25]: Th1 cells which are distinguished from Th2 cells by interferon-γ and Fas ligand expression [26] and initiate cell-mediated immunity by activating macrophages, but are relatively poor in B cell help, and Th2 cells which secrete IL-4, do not express fas ligand, and are effector helper cells for B cells. It is very unlikely that fas-ligand expressing Th1 cells foster fas-expressing germinal center B cell proliferation. What signals ensure that germinal center T cells deliver the right help?

There is good evidence that IL-12 plays a key role in regulating differentiation to the Th1 phenotype [25]. Dendritic cells produce IL-12 when activated through CD40 and therefore would be expected to induce Th1 cell priming. During immune responses to most infectious pathogens both Th1 and Th2 CD4+ cells play an effective role in immunity and clearly it is appropriate to generate the right help in each microenvironment. It is known that IL-4 promotes Th2 differentiation, but I think it unlikely that this is the initial signal as IL-4-deficient mice make virtually normal B cell responses and have germinal centers [27]. What on B cells might subvert this Th1 pathway?

The idea that B cells in some way induce help for their own responses is not new [25]. Recent evidence in favor of this idea is the failure of transgenic T cells to help B cells [22]. The reason for this was that all T cells primed in the host were Th1 in phenotype. Although an alternative explanation has been proposed for these results [28], they suggest B cells evoke Th2 help. One idea is that CD40 on B cells signals T cells through CD40 ligand [29]. However, as CD40 is widely expressed on other cells such as macrophages which typically evoke Th1 responses, this direct signaling effect seems unlikely to be the sole explanation.

Expression of New CD40 Family Member Molecules on B Cells Activated through CD40 Which Might Guide T Cells to Help B Cells

There are at least three different molecules expressed by CD40-activated B cells which might play a key role in directing the appropriate T cell help. (1) Germinal center B cells express B7 family members (probably post-CD40 activation

[30]) like other APCs. Blocking costimulation through CD28 abrogates germinal center development [14], and injection of anti-CD86 mAb reduces somatic mutation and germinal center size [31]. There is some suggestion that CD80 and CD86 may have differential effects on priming for Th1 and Th2 cells, respectively [32, 33]. Although their expression varies temporally, both B7 molecules are widely expressed on both dendritic cells and B cells, which would make differential priming by B cells and dendritic cells difficult to explain if this were the sole molecular explanation. (2) At a particular phase of germinal center development, B cells express CD27 ligand [34]. Like CD28, CD27 is expressed by the majority of T cells and costimulates T cell proliferation in vitro but whether there are distinct costimulatory properties is unknown [35]. (3) OX40-ligand is expressed by CD40-activated B cells [36], and its ligand OX40, in the CD40 family of receptors, is expressed by activated T cells. There is recent evidence that this molecule regulates B cell differentiation to class-switched plasma cells [37].

B Cell Proliferation within Germinal Centers and the Regulation of Somatic Mutation

Generating high affinity antibodies requires two components: efficient selection coupled with the ability to generate somatic mutants. Follicular dendritic cells (FDCs) capture immune complexes, and form an extensive surface area on which this selection can occur. Little is known of the function of accessory molecules on FDCs except the complement receptor complex appears to act like CD4/CD8 coreceptors on T cells [38]. CD19-deficient mice lack germinal centers and this could be related to either deficient signaling through the CD19/CD21/Ig receptor complex or alternatively deficient development of the follicular microenvironment [39, 40]. Also mice which lack lymphotoxin and type 1 but not type 2 TNF receptors lack germinal centers [41] although this may be due to developmental defects in secondary lymphoid organs.

Somatic mutants are rare in the preimmune repertoire, and rapidly accumulate in germinal centers. The key question is whether somatic mutation is linked with germinal center proliferation or regulated independently. Because high affinity variants which are better than the parent antibody are rare, theory predicts the most efficient strategy is one where cyclic bursts of high rate somatic mutation are coupled with selection and rapid clonal expansion without further mutation [42]. The reason that this strategy works best is that it generates the maximum number of mutants without risking loss of the rare variants which have better affinity.

Much of the evidence on germinal center proliferation is consistent with this theory. The initial B cell proliferation seen within B cell follicles is clonal and progeny are not mutated (this is the first phase of selection at the germline level)

[43]. At some point, perhaps when these follicular proliferations reach a certain size (1,000 cells), they form mature germinal centers with a dark zone of mutating centroblasts and a light zone where surface immunoglobulin-positive centrocytes undergo selection by antigen on FDCs in association with T cells. The abrupt appearance of somatic mutants is consistent with a switch, mimicking the burst of mutation that theory predicts.

The low frequency of improved antigen-binding variants make somatic mutation a high risk strategy. To shorten these odds, mutations are targeted to antigen-binding regions of the variable regions [44]. This means that a large number of binding variants may be generated with relatively few somatic mutations.

If mutation and proliferation were inextricably linked once the mutator was on, it would be easy to lose good mutants by accumulating further bad mutations in mutating progeny. It is more efficient to expand without further mutation until the clone size is large enough to support another round of mutation and selection. Therefore the ideal situation is if the mutation is regulated independently of proliferation.

Another less obvious reason why cyclic onset of mutation is a more efficient way to generate mutants is that selection only has to operate after the burst of mutation, rather than after each division (mutation without selection in a proliferating population risks loss of rare beneficial mutants). Centroblasts have a cell cycle time of 7 h [45], and pulse chase experiments indicate that they go on to become centrocytes [46]. Selection in the light zone of centrocytes takes around 20 h, which implies that many centroblasts in the dark zone are going through several divisions before they eventually differentiate to centrocytes, otherwise the germinal center reaction could not be sustained (renewal of centroblasts would be much slower than their exit to centrocytes). Given that it does not make sense to have mutation without selection it would seem sensible if selected B cells could expand as centroblasts without mutation which was switched on just prior to differentiation to centrocytes and subsequent selection.

What Kind of Molecular Mechanism Might Cause Oscillating Bursts of Mutation and Proliferation?

There is excellent evidence that CD40 activation plays the primary role in sustaining B cell proliferation within germinal centers. Both CD40 [47] and CD40 ligand [48] deficient mice lack germinal centers, somatic mutation and class-switched B cells, and injection of mAbs which block CD40 ligand reactions causes the rapid dissolution of germinal centers [31, 49].

A One Signal Model Where the Mutation Rate Is Separated from Proliferation

The simplest model is where B cells are driven to proliferate without mutation by CD40 ligand, but which become responsive to mutator signals. When CD40 ligand becomes limiting, mutation is switched on. A successful high affinity B cell derived from this cohort of mutating cells, by virtue of its improved capacity to capture and present antigen to T cells, would again get a CD40 ligand signal and expand clonally without further mutation at the expense of dying less successful B cells.

The Two-Signal Model Where Proliferation and Mutation Are Regulated by Separate Signals

Injection of blocking mAbs to CD40 ligand causes the rapid dissolution of germinal centers [31, 49], this is not associated with significantly increased apoptosis but with migration of B cells to the T zones and differentiation to antibody-producing cells. It seems that absence of CD40 signaling in the presence of other T cell signals promotes differentiation to plasma cells. From this it is clear that CD40 ligand-derived signals are important for sustaining proliferation within germinal centers.

Driving B cell proliferation through CD40 is not associated with mutation, either alone [50, 51] or in conjunction with anti-immunoglobulin signals. However, T cells in conjunction with anti-immunoglobulin do foster further mutation [51]. This suggests that there are two distinct signals for mutation, one dependent on immunoglobulin signaling, the other derived from T cells.

The mutation rate within germinal centers varies with the type of antigen and is correlated with the level of expression of CD86 on germinal center centrocytes [31, 52], the latter being induced by cross-linking surface immunoglobulin and CD40 signaling. Upregulation of CD86 may in turn evoke some mutator switch from germinal center T cells by signaling through CD28 or CTLA4. Presumably some antigens will differ in their capacity to upregulate CD86 on B cells, and this in turn would affect their capacity to evoke mutator signals from T cells. This would explain the lack of mutation in anti-CD86-treated mice [31], and the absence of germinal centers in mice where signaling through CD28 is blocked [14].

Other molecular interactions are also candidates. Anti-immunoglobulin signaling turns on CD27 expression, and this may make B cells responsive to CD27 ligand signals from T cells or from B cells themselves which express CD27 ligand after CD40 activation. CD27 ligand and its receptor [34] are expressed on the

---

immediate precursors of centroblasts, the IgD-positive CD38-positive population which is the earliest to show somatic mutation at a time when germinal center T cells are also expanding. Upregulation of CD27 by antigen retained on FDCs cross-linking immunoglobulin receptors might then provide the molecular signal to induce mutation when CD40 ligand signaling was limiting.

What Controls the Centrocyte Decision Point Which Determines Whether B Cells Become Memory B Cells or Centroblasts?

Centrocytes with useless receptors die by apoptosis due to lack of signaling. Reentry into the centroblast pathway is probably driven by CD40 ligand as anti-CD40 ligand antibodies lead to the rapid disappearance of germinal centers [31, 49]. In the competitive germinal center environment, only B cells with the highest affinity receptors would get a CD40 ligand signal. As it is important to rescue and expand rare mutants, it makes good sense that signaling through CD40 on B cells inhibits differentiation [53] and mutation [50].

It has been suggested that CD40 ligand can rescue centrocytes to become memory B cells [54, 55], but surprisingly blocking signaling through CD40 leads to little apoptosis but promotes B cell differentiation to antibody-producing cells [53, 55]. Quantitative differences in CD40 signaling could explain why some B cells become memory B cells and others become centroblasts. Alternatively there may be distinct molecules which direct cells into the memory pathway. Recently nerve growth factor, yet another member in the CD40 family of receptors [56], has been shown to selectively favor memory B cell survival. CD27 is also present on a subpopulation of human blood B cells which appear to be postantigen selection in that they have accumulated somatic mutations [57, 58], and recall memory responses can be evoked from these B cells. The role of this molecule in memory B cell formation is at present unknown.

Generation of Antibody-Producing Cells

Many centrocytes leave the germinal center and become antibody forming cells. Withdrawal of CD40 ligand is associated with plasma cell differentiation in vitro, and again both CD27 [59, 60] and OX40 signaling have been implicated in this pathway [36, 37]. Within germinal centers there may be distinct microenvironments which foster antibody production as distinct from memory B cell formation. It has been observed that memory T cells display heterogeneity in CD40 ligand expression, and this in itself might explain why some B cells become plasma cells and others proliferate. It seems likely that the mutator is switched off at this stage as neoplastic plasma cells from patients with myeloma have identical patterns of somatic mutations.

Although some B cells which leave germinal centers become antibody-producing cells, during both primary and secondary responses the great majority of antibody-forming precursors are derived from B cells proliferating in the T zones. OX40, which is expressed by activated T cells, is predominantly expressed in the T zones and may play an important role in inducing OX40 ligand expressing B cells to differentiate to switched plasma cells [37]. Soluble bivalent OX40 will mimic the T cell signal to B cells, suggesting in this example that the so-called receptor signals through the ligand.

Recall of Memory B Cell Responses

Memory and primary B cells appear to have different activation requirements. Memory B cells migrate to distinct locations, the marginal zone of spleen [61] and the interfollicular areas of lymph node [62], where they do not recirculate, but are ideally situated to be reactivated by antigen entering in the afferent lymph or by the bloodstream in the marginal sinus of spleen. It is not known what molecular mechanism retains B cells at these locations, but the B cell adhesion molecule, CD22, is one candidate. CD22 recognizes carbohydrate structures present on a protein backbone, and can bind macrophages [63]. Cross-linking CD22 on B cells primes them for activation through surface immunoglobulin [64] by sequestering the tyrosine phosphatase, PTP-1C [65]. This could explain why marginal zone B cells appear to be preactivated and so readily recruited into immune responses [46].

Conclusion

The effective generation of high affinity antibodies requires the clonal expansion of antigen-specific primary B cells, the generation of somatic mutants and their subsequent selection and differentiation into memory B cells and plasma cells. This B cell program is regulated by T cells and accessory cells which express costimulatory molecules guiding B cell development at particular stages. T cells reciprocally receive costimulatory signals from B cells which ensures that this process continues in a coordinated manner. In particular, it seems members of the CD40 family of receptors and ligands play a crucial role.

Acknowledgments

I would like to thank Ton Rolink and Fiona McConnell for their helpful criticisms on the manuscript. The Basel Institute was founded and is supported by F. Hoffmann-La Roche Ltd. Co., Basel, Switzerland.

References

1   Hoogenboom HR, Marks JD, Griffiths AD, Winter G: Building antibodies from their genes. Immunol Rev 1992;130:41–68.
2   Winter G, Griffiths AD, Hawkins RE, Hoogenboom HR: Making antibodies by phage display technology. Annu Rev Immunol 1994;12:433–455.
3   Steinman RM: The dendritic cell system and its role in immunogenicity. Annu Rev Immunol 1991; 9:271–296.
4   Cella M, Scheidegger D, Palmer-Lehman K, Lane P, Lanzavecchia A, Alber G: Ligation of CD40 on dendritic cells triggers production of high levels of interleukin-12 and enhances T cell costimulatory capacity: T-T help via APC activation. J Exp Med, in press.
5   Grewal IS, Xu J, Flavell RA: Impairment of antigen-specific T-cell priming in mice lacking CD40 ligand. Nature 1995;378:617–619.
6   Epstein MM, Di Rosa F, Jankovic D, Sher A, Matzinger P: Successful T cell priming in B cell-deficient mice. J Exp Med 1995;182:915–922.
7   Linsley PS, Greene JL, Tan P, Bradshaw J, Ledbetter JA, Anasetti C, Damle NK: Coexpression and functional cooperation of CTLA-4 and CD28 on activated T lymphocytes. J Exp Med 1992;176: 1595–1604.
8   Linsley PS, Ledbetter JA: The role of the CD28 receptor during T cell responses to antigen. Annu Rev Immunol 1993;11:191–212.
9   Tivol EA, Borriello F, Schweitzer AN, Lynch WP, Bluestone JA, Sharpe AH: Loss of CTLA-4 leads to massive lymphoproliferation and multiorgan tissue destruction, revealing a critical negative regulatory role of CTLA-4. Immunity 1995;3:541–547.
10 Waterhouse P, Penninger J, Timms E, Wakeham A, Shahinian A, Lee KP, Thompson CB, Griesser H, Mak TW: Lymphoproliferative disorders with early lethality in mice deficient in CTLA-4. Science 1995;270:985–988.
11 Ronchese F, Hausmann B, Hubele S, Lane P: Normal T cell priming to a protein antigen in mice transgenic for soluble CTLA-4. J Exp Med 1994;179:809–817.
12 Green JM, Noel PJ, Sperling AI, Walunas TL, Gray GS, Bluestone JA, Thompson CB: Absence of B7-dependent responses in CD28-deficient mice. Immunity 1994;1:501–508.
13 Shahinian A, Pfeffer K, Lee KP, Kundig TM, Kishihara K, Wakeham A, Kawai K, Ohashi PS, Thompson CB, Mak TW: Differential T cell costimulatory requirements in CD28-deficient mice. Science 1993;261:609–612.
14 Lane P, Burdet C, Hubele S, Scheidegger D, Müller U, McConnell F, Kosco-Villbois M: B cell function in mice transgenic for mCTLA4- H gamma 1: Lack of germinal centers correlated with poor affinity maturation and class switching despite normal priming of CD4+ T cells. J Exp Med 1994;179:819–830.
15 Cohen PL, Eisenberg RA: Lpr and gld: Single gene models of systemic autoimmunity and lymphoproliferative disease. Annu Rev Immunol 1991;9:243–269.
16 Singer GG, Abbas AA: The fas antigen is involved in peripheral but not thymic deletion of T cells in T cell receptor transgenic mice. Immunity 1994;1:365–371.
17 Smith KG, Nossal GJ, Tarlinton DM: FAS is highly expressed in the germinal center but is not required for regulation of the B-cell response to antigen. Proc Natl Acad Sci USA 1995;92:11628–11632.

18 Lane P, Haller C, McConnell F: Evidence that induction of tolerance in vivo involves active signaling via a B7 ligand-dependent mechanism: CTLA4-Ig protects Vβ8+ T cells from tolerance induction by the superantigen staphylococcal enterotoxin B. Eur J Immunol 1996;26:858–862.

19 Vyth Dreese FA, Dellemijn TA, Majoor D, de Jong D: Localization in situ of the costimulatory molecules B7.1, B7.2, CD40 and their ligands in normal human lymphoid tissue. Eur J Immunol 1995;25:3023–3029.

20 Marengere LEM, Waterhouse P, Duncan GS, Mittrücker H, Feng G, Mak TW: Regulation of T cell receptor signaling by tyrosine phosphatase SYP association with CTLA-4. Science 1996;272:1170–1173.

21 Jacobsen BA, Panka DJ, Nguyen K, Erikson J, Abbas AK, Marshak-Rothstein A: Anatomy of autoandibody production: Dominant localization of antibody-producing cells to T cell zones in Fas-deficient mice. Immunity 1995;3:509–519.

22 Stockinger B, Zal T, Zal A, Gray D: B cells solicit their own help from T cells. J Exp Med 1995;183:891–899.

23 Rathmell JC, Cooke MP, Ho WY, Grein J, Townsend SE, Davis MM, Goodnow CC: CD95 (Fas)-dependent elimination of self-reactive B cells upon interaction with CD4+ T cells. Nature 1995;376:181–184.

24 Jacob J, Kassir R, Kelsone G: In situ studies of the primary immune response to (4-hydroxy-3-nitrophenyl)acetyl. I. The architecture and dynamics of responding cell populations. J Exp Med 1991;173:1165–1176.

25 Seder RA, Paul WE: Acquisition of lymphokine-producing phenotype by CD4+ T cells. Annu Rev Immunol 1994;12:635–673.

26 Stalder T, Hahn S, Erb P: Fas antigen is the major target molecule for CD4+ T cell-mediated cytotoxicity. J Immunol 1994;152:1127–1133.

27 Kopf M, Le-Gros G, Bachmann M, Lamers MC, Bluethmann H, Kohler G: Disruption of the murine IL-4 gene blocks Th2 cytokine responses. Nature 1993;362:245–248.

28 Mason D: The role of B cells in the programming of T cells for IL-4 synthesis. J Exp Med 1996;183:717–719.

29 van Essen D, Kikutani H, Gray D: CD40 ligand-transduced co-stimulation of T cells in the development of helper function. Nature 1995;378:620–623.

30 Ranheim EA, Kipps TJ: Activated T cells induce expression of B7/BB1 on normal or leukemic B cells through a CD40-dependent signal. J Exp Med 1993;177:925–935.

31 Han S, Hathcock K, Zheng B, Kepler TB, Hodes R, Kelsoe G: Cellular interaction in germinal centers. Roles of CD40 ligand and B7-2 in established germinal centers. J Immunol 1995;155:556–567.

32 Kuchroo VK, Das MP, Brown JA, Ranger AM, Zamvil SS, Sobel RA, Weiner HL, Nabavi N, Glimcher LH: B7-1 and B7-2 costimulatory molecules activate differentially the Th1/Th2 developmental pathways: Application to autoimmune disease therapy. Cell 1995;80:707–718.

33 Freeman GJ, Boussiotis VA, Anumanthan A, Bernstein GM, Ke XY, Rennert PD, Gray GS, Gribben JG, Nadler LM: B7-1 and B7-2 do not deliver identical costimulatory signals, since B7-2 but not B7-1 preferentially costimulates the initial production of IL-4. Immunity 1995;2:523–532.

34 Lens SMA, Keehnen RMJ, Van Oers MHJ, van Lier RAW, Pals ST, Koopman G: Identification of a novel subpopulation of germinal center B cells characterized by expression of IgD and CD70. Eur J Immunol 1996;26:1007–1011.

35 Hintzen RQ, de-Jong R, Lens SM, van-Lier RA: CD27: Marker and mediator of T-cell activation? Immunol Today 1994;15:307–311.

36 Stüber E, Neurath M, Calderhead D, Fell HP, Strober W: Cross-linking of OX40 ligand, a member of the TNF/NGF cytokine family, induces proliferation and differentiation in murine splenic B cells. Immunity 1995;2:507–521.

37 Stüber E, Strober W: The T cell-B interaction via OX40-OX40L is necessary for the cell-dependent. J Exp Med 1996;183:979–989.

38 Fearon DT, Carter RH: The CD19/CR2/TAPA-1 complex of B lymphocytes: Linking natural to acquired immunity. Annu Rev Immunol 1995;13:127–149.

39 Rickert RC, Rajewsky K, Roes J: Impairment of T-cell-dependent B-cell responses and B-1 cell development in CD19-deficient mice. Nature 1995;376:352–355.

40   Engel P, Zhou LJ, Ord DC, Sato S, Koller B, Tedder TF: Abnormal B lymphocyte development, activation, and differentiation in mice that lack or overexpress the CD19 signal transduction molecule. Immunity 1995;3:39–50.

41   Matsumoto M, Mariathasan S, Nahm MH, Baranyay F, Peschon JJ, Chaplin DD: Role of lymphotoxin and type 1 TNF receptor in the formation of germinal centers. Science 1996;271:1289–1291.

42   Kepler TB, Perelson AS: Cyclic re-entry of germinal center B cells and the efficiency of affinity maturation. Immunol Today 1993;14:412–415.

43   Jacob J, Kelsoe G: In situ studies of the primary immune response to (4-hydroxy-3-nitrophenyl)acetyl. II. A common clonal origin for periarteriolar lymphoid sheath-associated foci and germinal centers. J Exp Med 1992;176:679–687.

44   Betz AG, Neuberger MS, Milstein C: Discriminating intrinsic and antigen-selected mutational hotspots in immunoglobulin V genes. Immunol Today 1993;14:405–411.

45   Zhang J, MacLennan ICM, Liu Y-J, Lane PJL: Is rapid proliferation in B centroblasts linked to somatic mutation in memory B cell clones? Immunol Lett 1988;18:297–300.

46   Liu YJ, Zhang J, Lane PJ, Chan EY, MacLennan IC: Sites of specific B cell activation in primary and secondary responses to T cell-dependent and T cell-independent antigens. Eur J Immunol 1991;21:2951–2962.

47   Kawabe T, Naka T, Yoshida K, Suematsu S, Yoshida N, Kishimoto T, Kikutani H: The immune response in CD40-deficient mice: Impaired immunoglobulin class switching and germinal center formation. Immunity 1994;1:167–178.

48   Xu J, Foy TM, Laman JD, Waldschmidt TJ, Elsemore J, Noelle RJ, Flavell RA: Mice deficient for the CD40 ligand. Immunity 1994;1:423–431.

49   Foy TM, Laman JD, Ledbetter JA, Aruffo A, Claassen E, Noelle RJ: gp39-CD40 interactions are essential for germinal center formation and the development of B cell memory. J Exp Med 1994;180:157–163.

50   Galibert L, van-Dooren J, Durand I, Rousset F, Jefferis R, Banchereau J, Lebecque S: Anti-CD40 plus interleukin-4-activated human naive B cell lines express unmutated immunoglobulin genes with intraclonal heavy chain isotype variability. Eur J Immunol 1995;25:733–737.

51   Källberg E, Jainandunsing S, Gray D, Leanderson T: Somatic mutation of immunoglobulin V genes in vitro. Science 1996;271:1285–1289.

52   Miller C, Stedra J, Kelsoe G, Cerny J: Facultative role of germinal centers and T cells in the somatic diversification of IgVH genes. J Exp Med 1995;181:1319–1331.

53   Lane P, Burdet C, McConnell F, Lanzavecchia A, Padovan E: CD40 ligand independent B cell activation revealed by CD40-ligand deficient T cell clones: Evidence for distinct activation requirements for antibody formation and B cell proliferation. Eur J Immunol 1995;25:1788–1793.

54   Liu Y-J, Joshua DE, Williams GT, Smith CA, Gordon J, MacLennan ICM: Mechanism of antigen-driven-selection in germinal centres. Nature 1989;342:929–931.

55   Arpin C, Dechanet J, Van Kooten C, Merveille P, Grouard G, Briere F, Banchereau J, Liu YJ: Generation of memory B cells and plasma cells in vitro. Science 1995;268:720–722.

56   Torcia M, Bracci-Laudiero L, Lucibello M, Nencioni L, Labardi D, Rubartelli A, Cozzolino F, Aloe L, Garaci E: Nerve growth factor is an autocrine survival factor for memory B lymphocytes. Cell 1996;85:345–356.

57   Maurer D, Holter W, Majdic O, Fischer GF, Knapp W: CD27 expression by a distinct subpopulation of human B lymphocytes. Eur J Immunol 1990;20:2679–2684.

58   Maurer D, Fischer GF, Fae I, Majdic O, Stuhlmeier K, Von Jeney N, Holter W, Knapp W: IgM and IgG but not cytokine secretion is restricted to the CD27+ B lymphocyte subset. J Immunol 1992;148:3700–3705.

59   Kobata T, Jacquot S, Kozlowski S, Agematsu K, Schlossman SF, Morimoto C: CD27-CD70 interactions regulate B-cell activation by T cells. Proc Natl Acad Sci USA 1995;92:11249–11253.

60   Agematsu K, Kobata T, Yang FC, Nakazawa T, Fukushima K, Kitahara M, Mori T, Sugita K, Morimoto C, Komiyama A: CD27/CD70 interaction directly drives B cell IgG and IgM synthesis. Eur J Immunol 1995;25:2825–2829.

61   Liu Y-J, Oldfield S, MacLennan I: Memory B cells in T cell-dependent antibody responses colonize the splenic marginal zones. Eur J Immunol 1988;18:355–362.

62   Liu YJ, Barthelemy C, de Bouteiller O, Arpin C, Durand I, Banchereau J: Memory B cells from human tonsils colonize mucosal epithelium and directly present antigen to T cells by rapid up-regulation of B7-1 and B7-2. Immunity 1995;2:239–248.

63   Stamenkovic I, Seed B: The B-cell antigen CD22 mediates monocyte and erythrocyte adhesion. Nature 1990;345:74–77.

64   Pezzutto A, Dörken B, Moldenhauer G, Clark EA: Amplification of human B cell activation by a monoclonal antibody to the B cell-specific antigen CD22, Bp 130/140. J Immunol 1987;138:98–103.

65   Doody GM, Justement LB, Delibrias CC, Matthews RJ, Lin J, Thomas ML, Fearon DT: A role in B cell activation for CD22 and the protein tyrosine phosphatase SHP. Science 1995;269:242–244.

Peter Lane, Basel Institute for Immunology, Grenzacherstrasse 487, CH–4005 Basel (Switzerland)
Tel. 041-61-6051312, Fax 041-61-6051364, E-mail lane@bii.ch

Ferrarini M, Caligaris-Cappio F (eds): Human B Cell Populations.
Chem Immunol. Basel, Karger, 1997, vol 67, pp 14–26

....

Tracing Antigen-Driven B Cell Development in Humans

Yong-Jun Liu

Schering-Plough, Laboratory for Immunological Research, Dardilly, France

The life history of B lymphocytes and T lymphocytes shares many similar features. They derive from immature precursor cells and use similar genes and strategies to encode, assembly and select their surface antigen receptors. T cell development in the thymus involves a series of stringent positive and negative selection processes, which ensure (1) the generated T cell receptors to distinguish self and nonself antigen, and (2) the dependence on the recognition of self-MHC to respond to nonself antigens. B cell development within the bone marrow also involves a series of selection processes, which ensure the generated B cell antigen receptors to directly recognize nonself antigen without the involvement of self MHC. The current pictures of primary T cell and B cell lymphopoiesis in the thymus and bone marrow, respectively, are generated by two kinds of experiments: (1) cell subset at each stage of gene rearrangement and the selection have been isolated according to the expression pattern of surface molecules, and (2) each cell subset is localized within a particular anatomical subcompartment of the thymus or bone marrow. Thus the whole differentiation pathway appears to follow a specific migration pattern through different functional compartments of thymus or bone marrow, where they interact with different stromal cells/accessory cells. These two experimental approaches, together with the molecular cloning of the stage-specific genes should ultimately permit the isolation of the regulatory molecules which drive the cells from one differentiation stage to the next during the primary B and T cell developments.

The final stage of primary B cell development in the bone marrow (lymphopoiesis) is the generation of large numbers of mature B cells which carry sIgM and sIgD antigen receptors [1]. These naive B cells continuously migrate into the peripheral lymphoid tissues, passing through the T cell and interdigitating cell-rich extrafollicular areas where thery may die or pursue their journey into the primary follicles where they become incorporated into the peripheral B cell pool [2].

Peripheral lymphoid tissues provide basic structures to facilitate antigen trapping and interactions between lymphocytes and antigen-presenting cells. All peripheral lymphoid tissues are organized into at least two basic structures, a T cell-rich interfollicular area and a B cell-rich follicle through which naive B cells percolate. The antigen-presenting cells within these two compartments are quite distinct: interdigitating dendritic cells of hematopoietic origin are mainly found in T cell-rich extrafollicular areas [3] and follicular dendritic cells (FDC) of mesenchymal origin are mainly localized in the B cell follicles [4–6]. In thymus-dependent humoral immune responses, antigen-specific naive B cells are firstly activated in extrafollicular areas in association with T cells and interdigitating dendritic cells. They undergo clonal expansion and differentiation either into short-lived plasma cells or germinal center (GC) founder cells [7, 8]. The activated B cell blasts colonizing the follicles undergo high rate proliferation yielding centroblasts that form the dark zones of GC [7–10]. Centroblasts undergo somatic mutation in their IgV region genes [11–15]. They give rise to nonproliferating centrocytes which undergo positive affinity selection in the light zone of GC [16]. FDC play a key role in B cell-positive selection through the immune complexes that they bind via Fc receptors as well as complement receptors. Then, high affinity centrocytes undergo isotype [17] switch and differentiation into either memory B cells or plasma cells [18–21].

Definition and Isolation of 7 B Cell Subsets from Human Tonsils

Specific markers have been identified during the past 2 decades that have allowed the identification of naive follicular mantle B cells and GC B cells on tissue sections and their subsequent isolation. In mice, naive follicular mantle B cells are sIgD+,PNAlow (peanut agglutinin binding low), while GC B cells are sIgD–,PNAhigh [22]. In humans, naive follicular mantle B cells are sIgD+,CD38–, while GC B cells are sIgD–,CD38+ [23]. These two subpopulations of B cells can be recognized both on tonsillar tissue sections (fig. 1A) and on the flow cytometry dot blot generated by a double anti-IgD and anti-CD38 staining (fig. 1B) [24]. In addition, two other B cell subpopulations composed of IgD+,CD38+ B cells and IgD–,CD38– B cells can be identified by flow cytometry analysis (fig. 1B). Three-color flow cytometry analysis of these four B cell subpopulations (fig. 1B) further shows that (1) the IgD+,CD38– follicular mantle B cell population contains a CD23– subset (Bm1) and a CD23+ subset (Bm2), (2) the IgD+,CD38+ B cell subpopulation contains an IgM+ subset (Bm2′) and an IgM– subset (Bm3δ), and

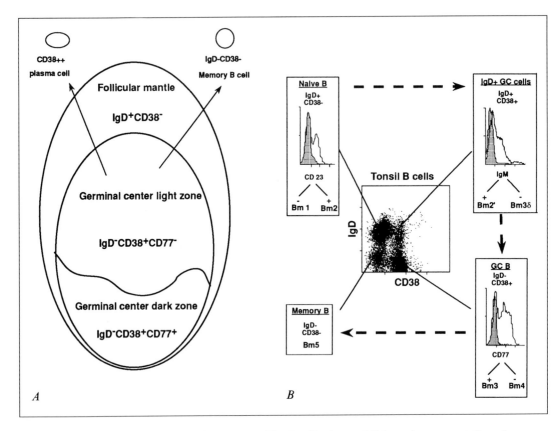

Fig. 1. Definition of human tonsillar B cell subsets. *A* Schematic representation of a tonsillar secondary follicle. It consists of a follicular mantle populated by IgD+,CD38– naive B cells and a GC populated by IgD–,CD38+ GC B cells. GC can be divided into a dark zone containing CD77+, Ki67+ centroblasts and a light zone containing CD77–,Ki67– centrocytes. In addition, CD38++ plasma cells can be found within both follicular and extrafollicular areas, while IgD–,CD38– memory B cells are mainly located within the intraepithelial area. *B* Tonsillar B cells can be sorted into 4 subsets based on anti-IgD and anti-CD38 double immunofluorescence staining. sIgD+,CD38– naive B cells can be further separated into a CD23+ subset (Bm1) and a CD23+ subset (Bm2), while sIgD+,CD38+ B cells can be further separated into an sIgM+ subset (Bm2') and a sIgM– subset (Bm3d). sIgD+,CD38+ GC B cells are separated into CD77+ centroblasts (Bm3) and CD77– centrocytes (Bm4). sIgD–,CD38– B cells (Bm5) represent memory B cells.

Table 1

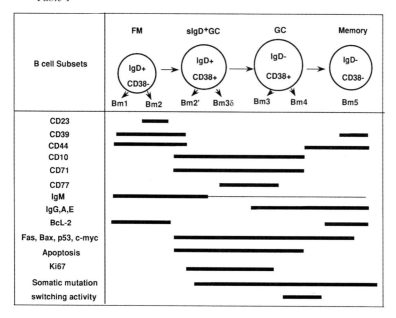

(3) the IgD–,CD38+ GC B cell subpopulation contains a CD77+ subset (Bm3) corresponding to the dark zone centroblasts and a CD77– subset (Bm4) corresponding to the light zone centrocytes. Accordingly, the IgD–, CD38– B cells displaying features of memory B cells was designated Bm5 [24]. The definition of B cell subsets permits us to determine the stages where proliferation, somatic mutation, programmed cell death and isotype switch take place within germinal centers.

sIgM+,IgD+,CD38+ GC Founder Cells Are Primed for Apoptosis before the Onset of Somatic Mutation [25]

sIgM+,IgD+,CD38+ B cells (Bm2′) most likely represent the transition stage during maturation of sIgD+,CD38– naive B cells (Bm1+2) to sIgD–,CD38+ GC B cells (Bm3+Bm4). Three-color flow cytometry in combination with in situ immunocytology and functional analysis shows that these sIgM+IgD+,CD38+ B cells have indeed acquired all the features of GC B cells (table 1): (1) they express all surface markers identified so far on GC B cells, including CD10 and CD71, (2) they express reduced levels of CD5, CD23 and CD44 markers expressed on follicular mantle B cells, (3) they express Fas/CD95 but no/or low bcl-2 protein, and undergo spontaneous apoptosis during culture, (4) about 30% of these cells express the proliferation-associated nuclear antigen ki67, and (5) they are localized within the GC. About 50% of the sIgM+,IgD+,CD38+ GC B cells contain germline immunoglobulin genes (0–2 mutations/sequences) [25]. Such a phenotype suggests the unmutated IgM+,IgD+,CD38+ B cells representing GC founder cells. Therefore, the genetic events underlying apoptosis are triggered before the onset of somatic mutation. Such an early triggering of the apoptosis program may contribute to the selection of unmutated GC B cells that have been observed in immunized mice [15] and humans [13]. Consequently, GCs may allow only B cells with relatively high affinity germline antigen receptors to undergo somatic mutation and affinity selection.

Overactivated Somatic Mutation in sIgM–,IgD+,CD38+ B Cells (Bm3δ) [26]

Isolated sIgM–,IgD+,CD38+ B cells display a typical centroblast phenotype (CD38+,Ki67+) and morphology (large lymphocytes with scanty pyroninophilic cytoplasm and blastic nucleus with multiple nucleoli). These cells express Fas/CD95 but not Bcl-2 and undergo rapid apoptosis in culture. Immunohistology demonstrates the localization of IgM–,IgD+,CD38+,Ki67+ within the dark zone of GC. Accordingly, this subset of B cells was named Bm3δ. Strikingly, these cells accumulated in their IgV genes the highest number of somatic mutations ever reported in normal B cells (average 40 mutations/sequence). This mutation frequency is 3-fold higher than that of the IgVH5-γ sequences of GC B cells from the same tonsils. The mechanism overactivating the somatic mutation machinery in these cells remains unclear. The high clonal relatedness frequently observed among sIgM–,IgD+,CD38+ B cell-derived δ-heavy chain sequences suggests that these cells originate from a few clones which have extensively proliferated within the GC dark zones. These cells may have undergone Cμ deletion through a homologous recombination between σμ and Σδ sequences [27–29], sequences located in the JH-μ intron and μ-δ intron, respectively. Such a recombination could remove (1) the switch region (Sμ) required for further isotype switch, (2) Cμ locus and (3) a putative somatic mutation silencer (SS), leading to an sIgM–,IgD+ phenotype and the overaccumulated somatic mutation. Such a deletion event may be triggered through the engagement of surface IgD antigen receptors by bacterial antigens, such as the IgD-binding protein D from *Haemophilus influenzae* B [30, 31] or by Fcδ receptors of T helper cells, a T cell subset known to enhance humoral immune responses [32]. In supporting this hypothesis, triggering sIgD only or sIgD together with sIgM may result in different effects on B cells, as sIgM but not sIgD is associated with prohibitin and a prohibitin-related protein that transduce negative cellular signals [33]. In keeping with this, it has been shown that the IgD-deficient mice are more sensitive to tolerance induction [34] and have a delay for affinity maturation during T cell-dependent antibody responses [35].

Within GC, the Isotype Switching Machinery Is Triggered after the Onset of Somatic Mutation [21]

Previous studies have demonstrated that somatic mutation and isotype switch are two independent processes [36]. An isotype switch can occur without somatic mutation, particularly during the B cell activation within the T cell-rich extrafollicular zones of the secondary lymphoid tissues [30]. The identification of somatically mutated sIgM+,IgD,–CD38+ [14, 37] and sIgM+,CD38+ B cells [25] indicates that somatic mutation can occur without an isotype switch as well. However, the majority of tonsillar GC B cells and memory B cells are found to express IgG or IgA [24], suggesting that isotype switching has occurred in most mutated B cells. To determine whether somatic mutation and isotype switching are triggered simultaneously or sequentially, the expression of immunoglobulin-sterile transcripts and the generation of extrachromosomal circular DNA were analyzed [21]. It was previously demonstrated that the expression of sterile transcripts is essential for the induction of isotype switching [38–40]. The generation of a primary sterile transcript is initiated at the I exon, located upstream of the S region. Following processing of primary transcript, the I exon is accurately spliced to the corresponding CH region. An isotype switching recombination is a process that moves the variable heavy chain segment (VDJ) to associate with a different constant (CH) region. This is mediated (with the exception of IgD) by the homologous recombination between switch regions (S regions), which are arrays of short tandem repeats, located 5′ of each constant region [41–43]. It leads to the formation and the excision of DNA circles, resulting in an intramolecular deletion of intervening CH genes. Therefore, sterile transcripts and switching DNA circles represent two molecular markers for isotype switching activity. The most abundant 5′Sγ-Sμ3′ DNA switching circles detected within GC B cells indicate that GC are the major site of isotype switch within human tonsils. The selective detection of sterile transcripts within GC centrocyte (Bm4) further suggests that the isotype switch occurs mainly within the GC light zone centrocytes after somatic mutation has been triggered within the GC dark zone centroblasts (Bm3). Somatic mutation and isotype switch seem to be regulated by two independent processes and the isotype switch does not terminate somatic mutation [36]. The physiological advantage of having isotype switching following affinity maturation by somatic mutation may be to avoid autoreactive B cells or low affinity B cells to acquire different Ig isotypes, which confers novel effector functions. Furthermore, the detection of isotype switching activity within centrocytes (Bm4) fits with their colocalization with a subset of T cells within the light zone of GC. This subset of T cells express CD40 ligand [44, 45] and secrete IL-4 and IL-10 [46], which represent key switching factors.

Human GC B Cells Are Primed for Apoptosis by c-myc, P[53], Fas, Bax in the Absence of Bcl-2 [47]

During T cell-dependent antibody responses, B cells within GC alter the affinity of their antigen receptor by introducing somatic mutations into IgV region genes. During this process, GC B cells are destined to die unless positively selected by antigens and CD40 ligands. To understand the survival/death control of GC B cell, the expression of four apoptosis-inducing genes, Fas, c-myc, BAX and P[53], together with the survival gene bcl-2 have been analyzed among the five tonsillar B cell subsets, including IgD+,CD38– naive B cells [CD23– (Bm1) and CD23+ (Bm2), IgD–,CD38+,CD77+ GC centroblast (Bm3), IgD–,CD38–, CD77– GC centrocyte (Bm4) and IgD–,CD38– memory B cell subset (Bm5 subset)]. We show that bcl-2 expression was only detectable with naive (Bm1 and 2) and memory B cell (Bm5) subsets; all four apoptosis-inducing genes were most importantly expressed within GC B cells. While Fas was equally expressed in centroblasts (Bm3) and centrocytes, Bax was more importantly expressed in centrocytes (Bm4) than in centroblasts (Bm3) and memory B cells (Bm5). c-myc, a positive regulator of the cell cycle was more importantly expressed in proliferating centroblasts (Bm3 subset) than in centrocytes (Bm4) and memory B cells (Bm5), while P[53], a negative regulator of the cell cycle, was more importantly expressed in nonproliferating centrocytes (Bm4 subset). The present result indicates that the survival/death of GC B cells are regulated by multiple genes and the expression of c-myc and P[53] in the absence of bcl-2 may prime the proliferating centroblasts (Bm3) and nonproliferating centrocytes (Bm4) to apoptosis.

Memory B Cells from Human Tonsils Colonize Mucosal Epithelium and Directly Present Antigen to T Cells by Rapid Upregulation of B7.1 and B7.2 [24]

IgD–,CD38– B cells can be isolated through negative selection, by depleting IgD+ B cells and CD38+ B cells, using either FACS sorting or magnetic beads. These cells express neither the GC markers CD10, CD71 and CD77 nor the follicular mantle B cell markers CD5 and CD23. All of them express CD20, CD39,

CD44, a large proportion express high levels of sIgG and only a few display sIgA. They do not express the proliferation-related nuclear Ki67 antigen, thus indicating their resting status. All express Bcl-2, only a few have low levels of Fas and, accordingly, they do not undergo rapid spontaneous apoptosis during in vitro culture. Upon polyclonal activation in vitro with IL-2, IL-10 and CD40 ligand, these cells, isolated from tetanus toxoid-vaccinated donors, produce large amounts of antitetanus toxoid IgG antibodies, while IgD+,CD38− naive B cells do not. Sequence analysis of their IgVH genes shows that they have undergone somatic muation [14]. These properties qualify these sIgD−,CD38− tonsillar B cells as memory B cells.

Human tonsillar memory B cells have two unique features. First, immuno-histological analysis shows that IgD−,CD38− memory B cells are mainly located within the mucosal epithelium but not in the follicles. Second, memory B cells but not naive B cells can induce proliferation of allo-CD4+ T cells, indicating that memory B cells can present antigen directly to T cells. The difference in the capacity of antigen presentation between memory B cells and naive B cells is associated with the rapid upregulation of B7.1 and B7.2 on memory B cells during the cognate interaction with the allospecific T cell line. Thus, the epithelial localization and the potent antigen-presenting capacity of memory B cells may explain the rapid and robust secondary humoral immune responses.

Plasma Cells from Human Tonsils Undergo Rapid Apoptosis, unless Rescued by Bone Marrow Stromal Cells [48]

Plasma cells represent the final stage of B cell differentiation. Because of their high level of CD38 expression [23], plasma cells can be isolated by sorting CD38++,CD20− cells from tonsillar populations that have previously been enriched in plasma cells through BSA gradients (fig. 2). CD38++,CD20− plasma cells express CD19, CD40, CD24, CD37, CD39, CD74 and HLA-DR. They do not express CD3, CD14, CD28, CD49d, CD56 and HLA-DQ. The purified CD38++,CD20− cells have a typical morphology of plasma cells, contain high levels of intracellular Ig, and release IgF and IgA in roughly equivalent levels. During in vitro culture, these plasma cells undergo rapid apoptosis, unless cultured on bone marrow stromal cells. The bone marrow stroma permits the survival of plasma cells through cell-cell interactions that are presently uncharacterized.

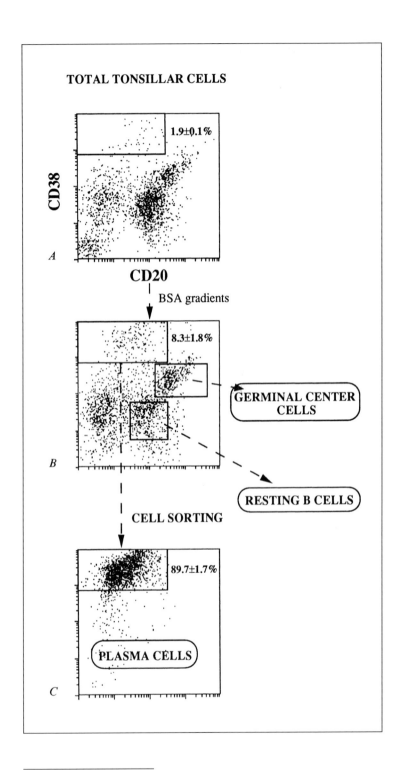

Generation of Memory B Cells and Plasma Cells in vitro [20]

The final step of GC B cell development is the differentiation of high affinity GC B cells towards memory B cells and plasma cells. Using CD38 and CD20, the molecular controls of differentiation of CD38+,CD20+ GC B cells into CD38−, CD20+ memory B cells and CD38+,CD20− plasma cells were analyzed in vitro.

First, GC B cells were cultured on CD40 ligand-transfected L cells with IL-2 and IL-10 to mimic the in vivo situation when high affinity GC B cells have picked up antigen from FDC [49] and are presenting it to CD40 ligand expressing GC T cells [44, 45]. GC B cells are rescued from apoptotic cell death [16], grow in exponential phase after 3 days of culture [50, 51] and do not acquire either CD38+,CD20− plasma cell phenotype or CD38−,CD20+ memory B cell phenotype.

After a further 4 days of culturing on CD40 ligand-transfected L cells with IL-2 and IL-10, these CD38+,CD20+ B blast cells acquire a CD38−,CD20+ memory B cell phenotype. They secrete little Ig and have the ability to proliferate in response to triggering through antigen receptor and CD40. In the absence of CD40 ligand, CD38+,CD20+ B blasts become terminally differentiated plasma cells after a 4-day culture with IL-2 and IL-10. This experiment reveals the central role of CD40 ligand in directing GC B cells toward the memory B cell pathway rather than the plasma cell pathway [20, 52, 53].

Conclusion

The phenotypic, functional and genetic characterization of human tonsillar B cell subsets (summarized in table 1) indicates that the apoptosis program, proliferation, somatic mutation and isotype switch are sequentially triggered within GC during T cell-dependent humoral immune responses. These highly purified human peripheral B cell subsets provide critical material to identify the triggers, the receptors and the internal signal transduction pathways that control the GC development.

Fig. 2. Isolation of the CD38high,CD20low tonsillar plasma cells. Total tonsillar cells obtained either directly after tonsil digestion or after three centrifugations over a 1.5% BSA solution were stained with FITC-conjugated anti-CD20 (horizontal axis, log scale) and PE-conjugated anti-CD38 mAbs (vertical axis, log scale). CD38high,CD20low plasma cells *(C),* CD38low,CD20medium resting B cells *(B)* and CD38medium,CD20high GC B cells *(A)* were stored with a FACStar plus®. Numbers indicate the percentages of cells contained in the corresponding inset (mean ± SEM of seven independent experiments).

Acknowledgments

I would like to thank S. Bonnet-Arnaud and M. Vatan for editorial assistance, and O. de Bouteiller, C. Arpin, P. Merville, J. Dechanet, I. Durand, C. Guret, F. Malisan, H. Martinez-Valdez, S. Lebecque, D. Capra, V. Pascual and J. Banchereau for their critical contribution and collaboration.

References

1   Melchers F, Haasner D, Grawunder U, Kalberer C, Karasuyama H, Winkler T, Rolink AG: Roles of IgH and L chains and of surrogate H and L chains in the development of cells of the B lymphocyte lineage. Annu Rev Immunol 1994;12:209–225.

2   MacLennan IC, Gray D: Antigen-driven selection of virgin and memory B cells. Immunol Rev 1986;91:61–85.

3   Steinman RM: The dendritic cell system and its role in immunogeneicity. Annu Rev Immunol 1991;9:271–296.

4   Nossal GJV, Abbot A, Mitchell J, Lummus Z: Antigens in immunity. Ultrastructural features of antigen capture in primary and secondary lymphoid follicles. J Exp Med 1968;127:277–290.

5   Tew JG, Kosco MH, Burton GF, Szakal AK: Follicular dendritic cells as accessory cells. Immunol Rev 1990;117:185–211.

6   Liu Y-J, Grouard G, de Bouteiller O, Banchereau J: Follicular dendritic cells and germinal centers. Int Rev Cytol 1996;166:139–179.

7   Liu Y-J, Zhang J, Lane PJL, Chan EY, MacLennan ICM: Sites of specific B cell activation in primary and secondary responses to T cell-dependent and T cell-independent antigens. Eur J Immunol 1991;21:2951–2962.

8   Jacob J, Kassir R, Kelsoe G: In situ studies of the primary immune response to (4-hydroxy-3-nitrophenyl) acetyl. I. The architecture and dynamics of responding cell populations. J Exp Med 1991;173:1165–1175.

9   Kroese FGM, Wubbena AS, Seijen HG, Nieuwenhuis P: Germinal centers develop oligoclonally. Eur J Immunol 1987;17:1069–1072.

10   Fliedner TM, Kress M, Cronkite EP, Robertson JS: Cell proliferation in germinal centre of the rat spleen. Ann NY Acad Sci 1964;113:578–588.

11   Jacob J, Kelsoe G, Rajewsky K, Weiss U: Intraclonal generation of antibody mutants in germinal centres. Nature 1991;354:389–392.

12   Berek C, Berger A, Apel M: Maturation of immune responses in germinal centers. Cell 1991;67: 1121–1129.

13   Küppers R, Zhao M, Hansmann M-L, Rajewsky K: Tracing B cell development in human germinal centres by molecular analysis of single cells picked from histological sections. EMBO J 1993;12: 4955–4967.

14   Pascual V, Liu Y-J, Magalski A, de Bouteiller O, Banchereau J, Capra JD: Analysis of somatic mutation in five B cell subsets of human tonsil. J Exp Med 1994;180:329–339.

15   McHeyzer-Williams MG, McLean MJ, Lalor PA, Nossal GJV: Antigen-driven B cell differentiation in vivo. J Exp Med 1993;178:295–307.

16   Liu YJ, Joshua DE, Williams GT, Smith CA, Gordon J, MacLennan ICM: Mechanisms of antigen-driven selection in germinal centers. Nature 1989;342:929–931.

17   Coico RF, Bhogal BS, Thorbecke GJ: Relationship of germinal centers in lymphoid tissue to immunologic memory. IV. Transfer of B cell memory with lymph node cells fractionated according to their receptors for peanut agglutinin. J Immunol 1983;131:2254–2257.

18   Klaus GGB, Humphrey JH, Kinkl A, Dongworth DW: The follicular dendritic cell: Its role in antigen presentation in the generation of immunological memory. Immunol Rev 1980;53:3–28.

19   Kosco MH, Burton GF, Kapasi ZF, Szakal AK, Tew JG: Antibody-forming cell induction during an early phase of germinal centre development and its delay with ageing. Immunology 1989;68:312.

20   Arpin C, Dechanet J, van Kooten K, Merville P, Grouard G, Brière F, Banchereau J, Liu Y-J: In vitro generation of memory B cells and plasma cells. Science 1995;268:720–722.

21   Liu YJ, Malisan F, de Bouteiller O, Guret C, Lebecque L, Banchereau J, Mills FC, Max EE, Martinez-Valdez H: Within germinal centers isotype switching of immunoglobulin genes occurs after onset of somatic mutation. Immunity 1996;4:241–250.

22   Rose ML, Birbeck MSC, Wallis VJ, Forrester JA, Davies AJS: Peanut lectin binding properties of germinal centres of mouse lymphoid tissue. Nature 1980;284:364–366.

23   Ling NR, MacLennan ICM, Mason D: B-cell and plasma cell antigens: New and previously defined clusters; in McMichael AJ (ed): Leucocyte Typing III. Oxford, Oxford University Press, 1987, pp 302–335.

24   Liu Y-J, Barthelemy C, de Bouteiller O, Arpin C, Durand I, Banchereau J: Memory B cells from human tonsils colonize mucosal epithelium and directly present antigen to T cells by rapid upregulation of B7.1 and B7.2. Immunity 1995;2:238–248.

25   Lebecque S, Arpin C, Banchereau J, Liu Y-J: Germinal center founder cells display propensity of apoptosis before onset of somatic mutation. J Exp Med, in press.

26   Liu Y-J, de Bouteiller O, Arpin C, Brière F, Galibert L, Ho S, Martinez-Valdez H, Banchereau J, Lebecque S: Normal human IgD+IgM− germinal center B cells can express up to 80 mutations in the variable region of their IgD transcripts. Immunity 1996;4:603–613.

27   Yuan D, Gilliam AC, Tucker PW: Regulation of expression of immunoglobulins M and D in murine B cells. Fed Proc 1985;44:2652–2659.

28   Yasui H, Akahori Y, Hirano M, Yamada K, Kurosawa Y: Class switch from μ to d is mediated by homologous recombination between Sμ and Sd sequences in human immunoglobulin gene loci. Eur J Immunol 1989;19:1399–1403.

29   Kluin PM, Kayano H, Zani VJ, Kluin-Nelemans HC, Tucker PW, Satterwhite E, Dyer MJS: IgD class switching; identification of a novel recombination site in neoplastic and normal B cells. Eur J Immunol 1995;25:3504–3508.

30   Janson H, Heden LO, Grubb A, Ruan MR, Forsgren A: Protein D, an immunoglobulin D-binding protein of *Haemophilus influenzae*: Cloning, nucleotide sequence and expression in *Escherichia coli*. Infect Immun 1991;59:119–125.

31   Forsgren A, Grubb AO: Many bacterial species bind human IgD. J Immunol 1979;122:1468–1472.

32   Coico RF, Siskind GW, Thorbecke GJ: Role of IgD and Td cells in the regulation of the humoral immune response. Immunol Rev 1988;105:45–67.

33   Terashima M, Kim K-M, Adachi T, Nielsen PJ, Reth M, Köhler G, Lamers MC: The IgM antigen receptor of B lymphocytes is associated with prohibitin and a prohibitin-related protein. EMBO J 1994;13:3782–3792.

34   Carsetti R, Köhler G, Lamers MC: A role of immunoglobulin D: Interference with tolerance induction. Eur J Immunol 1993;23:168–178.

35   Roes J, Rajewsky K: Immunoglobulin D (IgD)-deficient mice reveal an auxiliary receptor function for IgD in antigen-mediated recruitment of B cells. J Exp Med 1993;177:45–55.

36   Shan H, Shlomchik M, Weigert M: Heavy-chain class switch does not terminate somatic mutation. J Exp Med 1990;172:531–536.

37   Klein U, Küppers R, Rajewsky K: Variable region gene analysis of B cell subsets derived from a 4-year-old child: Somatically mutated memory B cells accumulate in the peripheral blood already at young age. J Exp Med 1994;180:1383–1393.

38   Coffman RL, Lebman DA, Rothman P: Mechanisms and regulation of immunoglobulin isotype switching. Adv Immunol 1993;54:229–270.

39   Sideras P, Mizuta T-R, Kanamori A, Suzuki N, Okamoto M, Kuze K, Ohno H, Doi S, Fukuhara S, Hassan MS, Hammarström L, Smith E, Shimizu A, Honjo T: Production of sterile transcripts of Cg genes in an IgM producing human neoplastic B cell line that switches to IgG-producing cells. Int Immunol 1989;1:631–642.

40   Xu L, Gorham B, Li SC, Bottaro A, Alt FW, Rothman P: Replacement of germ-line e promoter by gene targeting alters control of immunoglobulin heavy chain class switching. Proc Natl Acad Sci USA 1993;90:3705–3709.

41 Harriman W, Völk H, Defranoux N, Wabl M: Immunoglobulin class switch recombination. Annu Rev Immunol 1993;11:361–384.

42 Jung S, Rajewsky K, Radbuch A: Shutdown of class switch recombination by deletion of a switch region control element. Science 1993;259:984–987.

43 Radbruch A, Müller W, Rajewsky K: Class-switch recombination is IgG1 specific on active and inactive IgH loci of IgG1-secreting B-cell blasts. Proc Natl Acad Sci USA 1986;83:3954–3957.

44 Lederman S, Yellin MJ, Inghirami G, Lee JJ, Knowles DM, Chess L: Molecular interactions mediating T-B lymphocyte collaboration in human lymphoid follicles. Roles of T cell/B cell-activating molecule (5c8 antigen) and CD40 in contact-dependent help. J Immunol 1992;149:3817–3826.

45 Casamayor-Palleja M, Khan M: A subset of CD4+ memory T cells contains preformed CD40 ligand that is rapidly but transiently expressed on their surface after activation through the T cell receptor complex. J Exp Med 1995;181:1293–1301.

46 Butch AW, Chung G-H, Hoffmann JW, Nahm MH: Cytokine expression by germinal center cells. J Immunol 1993;150:39–47.

47 Martinez-Valdez H, Guret C, de Bouteiller O, Fugier I, Bancherau J, Liu YJ: Human germinal center B cells express the apoptosis inducing genes Fas, c-myc, P53 and Bax but not the survival gene bcl-2. J Exp Med 1996;183:227–236.

48 Merville P, Dechanet J, Desmoulière A, Durand I, de Bouteiller O, Garrone P, Banchereau J, Liu Y-J: Bcl-2 positive tonsillar plasma cells are rescued from prompt apoptosis by bone marrow fibroblasts. J Exp Med 1995;183:227–236.

49 Kosco MH, Szakal AK, Tew JG: In vivo obtained antigen presented by germinal center B cells to T cells in vitro. J Immunol 1988;140:354–360.

50 Bancherau J, de Paoli P, Vallé A, Garcia E, Rousset F: Long-term human B cell lines dependent on interleukin 4 and antibody to CD40. Science 1991;251:70–72.

51 Clark EA, Ledbetter JA: How B and T cells talk to each other. Nature 1994;367:425–428.

52 Lane P, Burdet C, McDonnel F, Lanzavecchia A, Padovan E: CD40-ligand-independent B cell activation revealed by CD40-ligand-deficient T cell clones: Evidence for distinct activation requirements for antibody formation and B cell proliferation. Eur J Immunol 1995;25:1788–1793.

53 Callard RE, Herbert J, Smith SH, Armitage RJ, Costelloe KE: CD40-cross-linking inhibits specific antibody production by human B cells. Int Immunol 1995;7:1809–1815.

Dr. Yong-Jun Liu, Schering-Plough, Laboratory for Immunological Research,
F–69571 Dardilly Cedex (France)
Tel. (33) 4 72 17 27 00, Fax (33) 4 78 35 47 50

Ferrarini M, Caligaris-Cappio F (eds): Human B Cell Populations.
Chem Immunol. Basel, Karger, 1997, vol 67, pp 27–44

....

T Cells in the Selection of Germinal Center B Cells

Montserrat Casamayor-Palleja, Adam Gulbranson-Judge,
Ian C.M. MacLennan

Department of Immunology, University of Birmingham Medical School,
Birmingham, UK

Germinal centers are sites where B cells undergo massive clonal expansion during T cell-dependent antibody responses [1, 2]. B cells in germinal centers activate a hypermutation mechanism that acts selectively on their immunoglobulin variable-region genes [3]. This can alter the B cells' affinity and specificity for the antigen that initiated the response. An antigen and T cell-dependent process exists that selects those B cells with high affinity for antigen to become plasma cells [4, 5] or memory B cells [6] – or to undergo further variable-region-directed hypermutation [7].

Germinal centers develop in B cell follicles; these are found in all secondary lymphoid tissues. A follicle not engaged in an immune response is known as a primary follicle; it contains small recirculating B cells that occupy the spaces in a network of follicular dendritic cells (FDC). An active transport mechanism exists that deposits antigen in the form of an immune complex on FDC [8] where it is retained for extended periods in a native form [9]. This FDC-associated antigen provides the only known long-term source of antigen in the body, other than that renewed by de novo synthesis – e.g. virus-infected cells and autoantigen. Antigen held on FDC is of the utmost importance to the processes that occur within germinal centers and has far-reaching influences on the development and maintenance of immune responses and immunological memory.

It is now clear that antigen-specific T cells also undergo clonal expansion in germinal centers (fig. 1) [10, 11]. These cells form a vital part of the selection of B cells that have mutated their immunoglobulin variable-region genes in germinal centers [12]. It is possible that T helper cells generated in germinal centers are important contributors to the pool of extrafollicular memory cells [11]; the num-

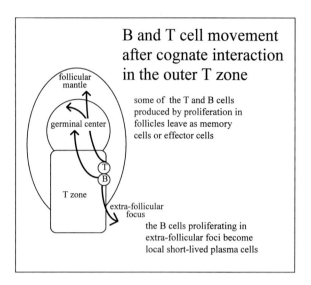

B and T cell movement after cognate interaction in the outer T zone

follicular mantle

germinal center

some of the T and B cells produced by proliferation in follicles leave as memory cells or effector cells

T zone

T
B

extra-follicular focus

the B cells proliferating in extra-follicular foci become local short-lived plasma cells

Fig. 1. Primed T cells migrate to the junction of the T zone and follicular mantle. B cells that have taken up antigen through their antigen receptors and have processed this also migrate to the T zone where they seek to make cognate interaction with primed T cells. Successful cognate interaction results in both the T cells and B cells migrating to sites of clonal expansion. Within the secondary lymphoid tissue T cells migrate to the follicle; activated B cells either migrate to extrafollicular foci in the red pulp, where this compartment abuts onto the T zone or to the follicles.

ber of T cells generated in follicles markedly exceeds the number seen to accumulate in follicles. Somatic mutations have been identified in the genes that encode the α-chain of T cell receptors [10] and it is likely that T cells with such mutations are selected in follicles – in this case on the basis of their affinity for processed antigen presented by follicular B cells. Clearly this would be associated with death of some T cells in situ; the proportion of the excess T cells that die in follicles and the fractions that are exported as memory or effector T cells have to be determined.

Germinal Center Formation

Germinal center formation is initiated following an antigen-specific interaction between primed T cells and B cells that have taken up and processed antigen. This occurs in T zones of secondary lymphoid tissues (fig. 1) [13]. Following this interaction the B cells start to proliferate and migrate from the T zone; some go to the follicles where they form germinal centers – others form proliferative foci in

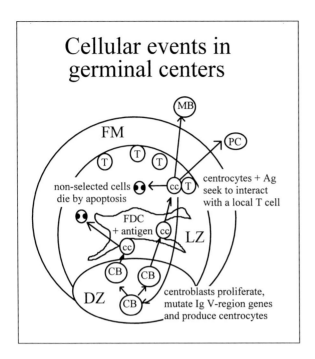

Cellular events in germinal centers

MB

FM

T T T

PC

non-selected cells ↶← cc T   centrocytes + Ag
die by apoptosis   seek to interact
                                      with a local T cell

FDC
+ antigen cc   LZ

cc

CB CB

DZ CB

centroblasts proliferate,
mutate Ig V-region genes
and produce centrocytes

Fig. 2. The proliferating B cells in germinal centers, centroblasts (CB), are located at one pole of the follicle in a compartment known as the dark zone (DZ). They continually give rise to nonproliferating cells, centrocytes (CC), that enter the FDC-rich light zone (LZ) where first they seek to pick up antigen from FDC. If this is successful they move to the outer rim of the light zone where they attempt to make cognate interaction with antigen-specific T cells; these are located particularly at the junction of the light zone with the follicular mantle (FM). Successful interaction with T cells leads to differentiation along one of 3 pathways: to centroblasts, to memory B cells (MB) or to plasma cells (PC) that have a life span of around 1 month. Centrocytes either failing to pick up antigen from FDC or failing to make cognate interaction with local T cells die in situ by apoptosis and are rapidly taken up by local macrophages.

the red pulp at its junction with the T zone. The B blasts in these extrafollicular foci differentiate after 3 days into short-lived plasma cells [14]. The T cells also migrate from the T zone; some may leave the secondary lymphoid organ but others pass into the follicles where they may proliferate – surprisingly they have not been seen to enter the extrafollicular foci of B cell proliferation [11]. T cell proliferation in the follicles is most marked in primary antibody responses. In secondary responses similar numbers of T cells enter the follicles but the rate of proliferation is much lower. This may reflect the recruitment of circulating memory cells into the follicles.

On average 2–3 B cells seed each follicle to form a germinal center; they undergo exponential growth and within 3 days fill the FDC network having increased in number to 10^4 to 1.5×10^4 cells [2]. The recirculating B cells are now confined to the periphery of the follicle where they form the follicular mantle. When the collection of B blasts fills the FDC network the compartmentalization develops which characterizes fully developed germinal centers (fig. 2). The proliferating B blasts then migrate to the pole of the follicle nearest to the T zone to form the dark zone. There the cells, now known as centroblasts, continue to proliferate but do not increase in number for they continually give rise to nondividing progeny known as centrocytes [2, 15]. Centrocytes come out of cell cycle and enter the FDC network which corresponds to the light zone of the germinal center. There they die by apoptosis unless they are positively selected to become memory B cells [6] or plasma cells [4] or to readopt a centroblast phenotype and presumably undergo further somatic mutation in the dark zone [7].

In mice the antigen-specific T cells that are induced to migrate to follicles are found both in the developing germinal center and the follicular mantle and proliferate in both sites [11]. As the germinal center compartmentalizes the T cells become concentrated at and near the junction of the follicular mantle and light zone. Antigen-specific T cell numbers decline as the germinal center reaction subsides 3–4 weeks after immunization, but some remain along with memory B blasts for long after the end of the germinal center response. These cells may be responsible for maintaining an output of memory B and T cells and plasma cells.

Selection of Germinal Center B Cells

Both the affinity and the specificity for antigen may alter as a result of hypermutation in germinal center lymphocytes. In theory self-reactive lymphocytes could be formed. Characteristically the nuclear debris from cells undergoing apoptosis (tingible bodies) is seen within germinal center macrophages. Fliedner [16] showed that this was derived from cells that have recently been in cell cycle. Although this is seen most easily in the dark zone, quantitative histology shows macrophages with apoptotic debris throughout the germinal center with the highest frequency of these cells in that part of the dense FDC network closest to the dark zone [17]. It was suggested that tingible bodies are the remnants of germinal center B cells that have mutated their immunoglobulin variable-region genes but have failed to obtain positive selection signals [18]. Evidence supporting this hypothesis was provided by the finding that freshly isolated germinal center B cells undergo apoptosis within a few hours if they are cultured at 37 °C. This effect could be delayed for several hours but not prevented by cross-linking the B cell surface antigen receptors with anti-Ig bound to sheep red blood cells [19]. This is consistent with the concept that interaction with antigen held on FDC is involved in centrocyte selection; this could not be the sole selection signal, for death was only averted for a short period. An extensive search for a second selection signal showed that ligation of CD40 expressed on the surface of B cells by monoclonal antibody (mAb) resulted in prolonged inhibition of apoptosis of the germinal center B cells [19]. The significance of this finding only became apparent with the identification of a natural ligand for CD40; it is a molecule induced on the surface of T cells when they are activated through their T cell receptor [20–23]. This suggested that centrocytes are first selected on the basis of their capacity to take up antigen held on the surface of FDC, to process this antigen and then present the resulting peptides to a local antigen-specific T cell. Successful cognate interaction results in the delivery of signals that inhibit apoptosis and induce differentiation (fig. 2). The rest of this review describes experiments that test the hypothesis that cognate interaction between T and B cells is required for cell selection in germinal centers; it probes the signals that may be delivered during this interaction.

Continuous CD40 Ligation of Germinal Center B Cells Is Unlikely to Occur in vivo and Does Not Result in Them Adopting a Memory B Cell Phenotype in vitro

Ligation of CD40 on human tonsil germinal center B cells in vitro with either CD40 mAb [19] or recombinant CD40 ligand [24] inhibits their tendency to enter apoptosis. After 48 h culture most of the resulting cells have come out of cell cycle – early experiments led to the suggestion on morphological grounds that these cells might represent memory B cells. This is not confirmed if their phenotype is compared with that of memory B cells freshly isolated from tonsil (fig. 3, 4). The phenotype of germinal center B cells isolated from human tonsil on the basis of their lack of surface CD39 and IgD expression [19] is shown in figure 3; they are CD38high, CD44low/–, CD77low/high and sIglow. Tonsil memory B cells by contrast are CD38–/low, CD44+, CD77– and sIghigh [25–28]. The phenotype adopted by germinal center B cells cultured with CD40 mAb is quite unlike either of these two populations or indeed any other tonsil B cell subset; it becomes CD44high, universally CD77high and sIghigh; CD38 expression is maintained [7]. A number of activation antigens are acquired – CD23, CD25, CD86 – that are not found or are sporadically expressed at low levels on germinal center or memory B cells (fig. 4). The acquisition of a nonphysiological phenotype has also been reported by other groups when they use short-term cultures with soluble CD40 mAb [29] or CD40 ligand transfected into fibroblasts as a feeder layer [30]. No differentiation towards Ig secreting cells was seen in 48-hour cultures of germinal center B cells in the presence of CD40 mAb and no Ig was secreted into these

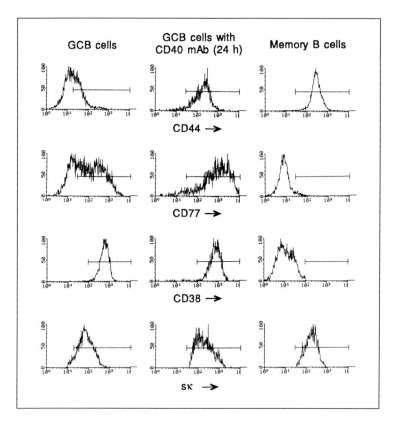

Fig. 3. The phenotype of freshly isolated germinal center B cells (GCB) compared to that of germinal center B cells cultured with soluble CD40 mAb for 24 h and freshly isolated memory B cells. This was assessed by double color immunofluorescence staining on the flow cytometer. Data correspond to viable lymphocyte-lymphoblast cell gate as determined by forward and 90° light scatter profiles and are representative of 10 experiments [adapted from 7].

cultures. The resulting B cells remained CD20+ and became sIghigh, which weighs against the cells differentiating towards plasma cells.

In longer-term cultures where germinal center B cells were cultured for 7 days with IL-2, IL-10 and CD40 ligand-transfected fibroblasts, a memory B cell phenotype was acquired [31]. The long time taken to generate memory B cells in this system is not consistent with the estimated tempo for centrocytes to differentiate to memory B cells in vivo. Hanna [15] as long ago as 1964 calculated that the transit time of centrocytes through the light zone of the germinal centers is in the order of 7 h. This is confirmed by the finding that memory B cells in the marginal

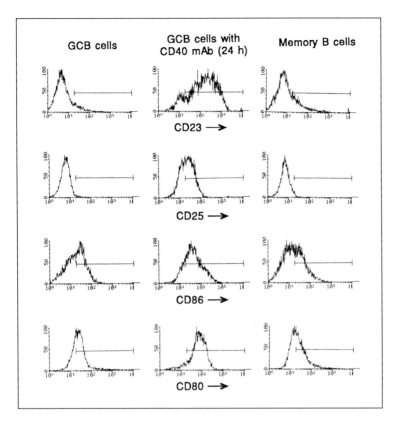

Fig. 4. Activation molecules expressed by germinal center B cells (GCB) cultured with soluble CD40 mAb. Expression of the activation molecules CD23, CD25, CD86 and CD80 was assessed on freshly isolated germinal center B cells, germinal center B cells cultured with soluble CD40 mAb for 24 h and freshly isolated memory B cells by single color flow cytometry. The histograms show events in the viable lymphocyte-lymphoblast cell gate as determined by forward and 90° light scatter profiles [adapted from 7].

zone of rats are not in cell cycle but can originate from proliferating cells – presumably centroblasts – within 12 h [32]. These findings indicate that in vivo, the time available for a centrocyte to make cognate interaction with a T cell is in the order of minutes to a few hours and certainly not days. Intuitively one would not expect CD40 ligand to be expressed in a stable fashion on the surface of germinal center T cells and the available data indicate that it is not. About half the T cells in human tonsil germinal centers contain preformed CD40 ligand and this can be rapidly but transiently expressed on the cell surface by cross-linking the T cell antigen receptors [33]. Yellin et al. [34] showed that induced CD40 ligand was

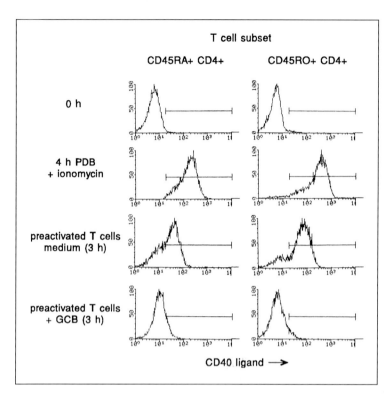

Fig. 5. Germinal center B cells (GCB) cause rapid downregulation of CD40 ligand expressed on the surface of autologous tonsil T cells. CD40 ligand expression was assessed on naive (CD45RA+ CD4+) and memory (CD45RO+ CD4+) T cells before (top row) and after 4 h of culture with phorbol dibutyrate (PDB) and ionomycin (second row). The preactivated T cells were then washed thoroughly and the CD40 ligand expression reassessed after 3 h culture in medium alone (third row) or with autologous germinal center B cells (bottom row). CD40 ligand expression was determined with single color immunofluorescence staining by flow cytometry with biotinylated M90 (anti CD40 ligand) mAb [adapted from 7].

rapidly downregulated from human blood T cells when they were cocultured with autologous blood B cells. This also happens when germinal center T cells are cocultured with autologous centrocytes (fig. 5) [7]. These data are consistent with the concept that centrocytes take up antigen from FDC, process this and then attempt to interact with T cells located at the light zone and follicular mantle junction. If specific interaction occurs CD40 ligand is expressed at the site of centrocyte contact with the T cell; the costimulus is delivered solely to the interacting centrocyte – the CD40 ligand is immediately withdrawn or shed and the centrocyte disengages. The next section describes experiments that test this possibility.

Transient CD40 Ligation Is Required but Is Not Sufficient for Germinal Center T Cells to Prevent Autologous Centrocytes Killing Themselves by Apoptosis

The transient T cell activation system of culture with phorbol dibutyrate and ionomycin used in the experiments depicted in figure 5 was used to induce CD40 ligand expression by tonsil CD45RA– and CD45RO– CD4+ T cells. These two subsets of T cells are largely nonoverlapping; the CD45RA– cells are CD45RO+ and comprise primed T cells, germinal center T cells and memory T cells. The CD45RO– cells are CD45RA+ – a characteristic of naive T cells [35]. Only about half the CD45RA– subset and none of the CD45RO– cells contain preformed CD40 ligand that can be rapidly expressed on their surface by cross-linking the T cell antigen receptor. On the other hand, after 4 h exposure to phorbol dibutyrate and ionomycin indistinguishable levels of CD40 ligand expression were seen on both CD45RA– and CD45RO– T cells. Both subsets downregulate CD40 ligand completely within 3 h on coculture with autologous germinal center B cells (fig. 5). Consequently the ligation of CD40 on the B cells in these cocultures is only transient. This transient CD40 ligand is not sufficient in itself to prevent centrocytes killing themselves by apoptosis; centrocytes cocultured with preactivated CD45RO– die as quickly as isolated centrocytes cultured in medium only. The preactivated CD45RO– T cells are not obviously killing the centrocytes for they do not express Fas ligand and do not kill cell lines susceptible to cytolytic T cell-mediated lysis. It seems likely, therefore, that the centrocytes simply die by default as they have not received a positive signal that rescues them entering apoptosis. By contrast autologous CD45RA– T cells with induced surface CD40 ligand expression rescue as many germinal center B cells from apoptosis as CD40 mAb (table 1). This rescue effect is dependent on CD40 ligation; inhibition of ligation with a blocking mAb prevents rescue. In conclusion, these experiments indicate that transient CD40 ligation alone is not sufficient for centrocyte rescue from apoptosis: additional and as yet unidentified signals must be delivered by the CD45RA– T cells to achieve rescue.

In parallel experiments to those shown in table 1 it was found that a small but statistically significant proportion of germinal center B cells (5–15%) survived when they were cocultured with nonpreactivated autologous CD45RA– T cells [7]. The surviving germinal center B cells may have been centrocytes that had taken up antigen from the FDC network, processed it and then presented peptides on their surface. As many or most of the germinal center T cells are specific for the antigens that induced the germinal center reaction [11, 36, 37] it is likely that a proportion of the autologous CD45RA– T cells are specific for peptides presented by autologous centrocytes. The rescue from apoptosis brought about by these T cells may result from true cognate interaction; it is dependent on CD40 ligand expression, for it is inhibited by CD40 ligand blockade [unpubl. data].

Table 1. Viability of germinal center B cells cultured with CD40 mAb or autologous T cells induced to express CD40 ligand on their surface

Tonsil cells used in coculture		Culture additive	GCB survival after 48 h, %
B cells	activated T cells[1]		
GCB	none	none	<5
GCB	none	CD40 mAb	≈50
GCB	CD45RO+ CD4+	none	≈50
GCB	CD45RO+ CD4+	blocking CD40L mAb	<5
GCB	CD45RA+ CD4+	none	<5

[1] Naive (CD45RA+ CD4+) and memory (CD45RO+ CD4+) T cells were preactivated with phorbol dibutyrate and ionomycin for 4 h before being added to autologous germinal center B (GCB) cells in a ratio 1 to 1. As shown in figure 5 culture with phorbol dibutyrate and ionomycin for 4 h induced high levels of surface CD40 ligand expression by both T cell subsets. The viability of germinal center B cells cultured in medium only, with CD40 mAb (1 μg/ml), or with autologous preactivated memory or naive T cells, was assessed as described [7]. M91, a CD40 ligand blocking mAb (15 μg/ml), was added to the cultures of germinal center B cells with autologous preactivated memory T cells at the start of the culture.

Preactivated Germinal Center T Cells Selectively Form Conjugates with the Centrocytes from Autologous Germinal Center B Cell Preparations and Induce Most of These to Adopt a Memory B Cell Phenotype within 24 h

On coculture germinal B cells and preactivated autologous T cells form elongated clumps of 10 cells or more across. The number of cells present in these conjugates is higher when the T cells are preactivated. Careful analysis of the phenotype of the germinal center B cells that form conjugates with autologous T cells has been carried out using flow cytometry and confocal microscopy. This indicates that centrocytes (CD44low, CD77low) rather than centroblasts (CD44–, CD77high) form conjugates [7]. After 3 h coculture at a 1 to 1 ratio CD44low, CD77low B cells colocalize on flow cytometry with the CD2+, CD3+ T cells. CD44–, CD77high cells do not form firm bonds with the T cells. Within 24 h, most of the B cells in the conjugates upregulate CD44 and sIg expression, become CD77low and remain CD23–, CD25– and CD38high (fig. 6). This is the phenotype of freshly isolated memory B cells, apart from the continued expression of CD38. As freshly isolated memory B cells cocultured with autologous memory T

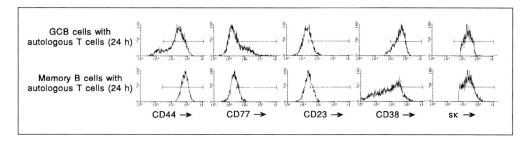

| | CD44 → | CD77 → | CD23 → | CD38 → | sκ → |

Fig. 6. The phenotype of germinal center B (GCB) cells cocultured with autologous memory T cells compared with that of memory B cells cocultured with memory T cells. Germinal center and memory B cells were cocultured with autologous memory T cells and the phenotype of the resulting B cells was assessed by double color FACScan staining. The data shown correspond to the phenotype of CD20+ cells for CD44, CD77, CD23 and CD38 and sκ for sκ+ cells [this figure has been taken from ref. 7].

cells also upregulate CD38 (fig. 6) the conclusion that memory B cells are being generated is still tenable.

One of the features that characterize germinal center B and T cells is the lack of Bcl-2 expression. Tonsil memory B cells express this protein that has an anti-apoptotic effect [38] indicating that selection of germinal center B cells is associated with reexpression of Bcl-2. CD40 ligand of germinal center B cells with soluble CD40 ligand induces reexpression of Bcl-2 on the surviving cells between 24 and 48 h of culture [24]; this is too slow a tempo to account for the prevention of apoptosis achieved through CD40 ligation – it seems likely that initial rescue from apoptosis is Bcl-2-independent, but the expression of this protein is required if these cells are to survive subsequently outside germinal centers. Preactivated memory T cells also induced Bcl-2 expression by cocultured centrocytes; a small subset starts to reexpress Bcl-2 within 24 h coculture – the majority become Bcl-2+ between 24 and 48 h after the cultures are initiated.

A Subset of Centrocytes Revert to a Centroblast-Like Phenotype on Coculture with Autologous Memory T Cells

The possibility of centrocytes reentering the dark zone to undergo further proliferation and somatic hypermutation was first suggested from mathematical studies [39]. Recent experiments in vivo from Kelsoe's group [40] have reopened this hypothesis. Blocking of CD40/CD40 ligand interactions in established germinal centers results in the dissolution of these structures [40]. If a proportion of centrocytes revert to centroblasts as a result of cognate interaction with local T cells, the blockade of these interactions is likely to result in the dissolution of germinal centers. The recent finding that B cells can express surface CD40 ligand when activated in vitro [41] has opened the possibility that centroblasts are a self-renewing population and that CD40 ligand on these cells acts as an autocrine stimulus. This result might explain the effects of CD40 ligand blockade on established germinal centers, but cannot counter the recent unpublished finding from Kelsoe's laboratory that established germinal centers are destroyed by antibodies against the T cell receptor complex. As there are vanishingly small numbers of T cells in the dark zone of germinal centers [42] the implication is that centroblasts are renewed by cells that have recently been under the influence of T cells. The ipsiclonal nature of the centrocytes and centroblasts in a single germinal center [2, 43] indicates that centrocytes are the only possible candidates for centroblast renewal.

While most centrocytes forming conjugates with autologous germinal center T cells adopt a memory B cell phenotype, a small subset of the centrocytes are induced to express high levels of surface CD77 and cease to express CD44 – the phenotype characteristic of centroblasts. This is apparent from detailed time course studies of the coculture of autologous germinal center T and B cells. As is set out above conjugates are selectively formed between T cells and centrocytes. The nonincorporated centroblasts die by apoptosis within the first 12 or so hours. In some experiments more centroblasts were found at 24 than 12 h after the start of coculture; in all experiments there were substantial numbers of centroblasts in the cocultures after 24 h, while none remained in cultures of germinal center B cells alone. Isolated centroblasts die more rapidly by apoptosis than centrocytes [28], which may reflect the high expression of c-Myc and lack of cytoplasmic Bcl-2 by centroblasts [44]. The reappearance of centroblasts between 12 and 24 h raises the possibility that some centrocytes that form conjugates with CD45RA– T cells are induced to readopt a centroblast phenotype; these reversional cells then dissociate from the conjugates and in the absence of dark zone stroma die.

The signals that induce germinal center B cells to differentiate to memory B cells or centroblasts in this system are still unresolved. The germinal center T cell population is heterogeneous; although germinal center T cells are CD45RO+, a proportion of these T cells are CD57+ and only about 50% of the germinal center T cells contain preformed CD40 ligand. It is possible that different germinal center T cell subsets cause centrocytes to differentiate to different cell types. It has been reported that CD4+ CD57– primed T cells induce B cells to proliferate or to secrete immunoglobulin while their CD57+ counterpart apparently do not [45, 46]. Evidence against CD57+ T cells being a distinct CD4+ germinal center T cell subset comes from the analysis of monoclonal leukemic cells from 3 patients with

CD4+, CD45RO+, cytoplasmic CD40 ligand+ neoplastic cells. In each of these cases about a third of these cells were CD57+ even after extended periods in culture [Casamayor-Palleja et al., unpubl. data].

Signalling through Protein Kinase C Might Be Involved in Memory B Cell Formation

The data shown in the previous two sections are consistent with physiological CD40 ligation being required to generate memory B cells but not being a sufficient signal to achieve this on its own; additional signals are needed. These signals seem to be provided by primed but not naive T cells. One of the possibilities is that these additional signals are provided by cytokines. Naive and primed T cells have been reported to have different cytokine profiles. Differences in their phenotypes have also been found. The T cell receptor on memory T cells associates with CD4 and CD45RO during T cell activation, while on naive T cells these three molecules act independently. Likewise, memory T cells express higher levels of the adhesion molecules CD11a, CD29, CD2 and CD44 [47], and bind more strongly to B7-1 and 2 and CD54 [48]. It is likely that adhesion molecules on memory T cells play a role in the rescue of centrocytes from apoptosis, but as CD40 ligand blockade inhibits the delivery of selection signals these adhesion molecule interactions do not furnish sufficient signals to achieve survival and subsequent differentiation.

Preliminary experiments with phorbol esters and the calcium ionophore ionomycin show that germinal center B cells can be rescued from entering apoptosis by these two reagents [49]; phorbol myristate acetate acts directly on the protein kinase C. Despite original findings that ligation of CD40 with CD40 mAb may act on some of the protein kinase C isoforms in tonsil resting B cells [50] the current consensus is that signal transduction through CD40 does not rely on protein kinase C. Activation of B cells with CD40 ligand-expressing plasma membranes of activated T cells did not result in protein kinase C translocation or phosphorylation of the endogenous protein kinase C substrate MARCKS [51, 52]. Furthermore activation of the transcription factor NF-κB [53] and the stress-activated protein kinase c-Jun [54] by CD40 ligation has been reported to be independent of protein kinase C.

Flow cytometry studies were carried out to see if germinal center B cell rescue from apoptosis induced by phorbol ester and ionomycin, unlike CD40 ligand, induces a physiological phenotype. The results of these studies are summarized in figures 7 and 8. The phenotype of germinal center B cells treated with CD40 mAb plus IL-4 or phorbol myristate acetate plus ionomycin was compared with that of memory B cells treated with the same agents. While the phenotypes of the germi-

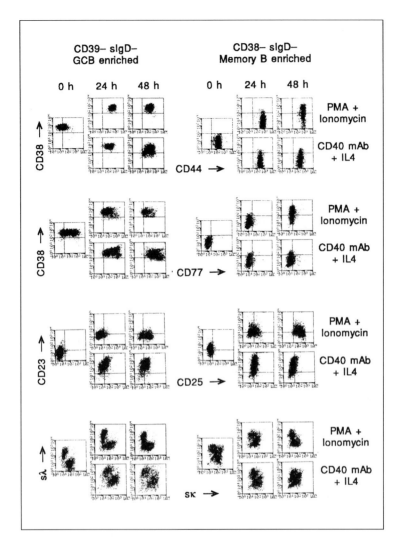

Fig. 7. Comparison of the phenotype of germinal center B cells (GCB) cultured with phorbol myristate acetate plus ionomycin with that of germinal center B cells cultured with CD40 mAb plus IL-4. Two-color FACScan dot plots showing phenotypic changes in germinal center B cells and memory B cells after 24 and 48 h culture with either phorbol myristate acetate (PMA) plus ionomycin or CD40 mAb with IL-4. The data shown are based upon the viable lymphocyte and blast cell gate determined by forward and 90° light scatter profiles.

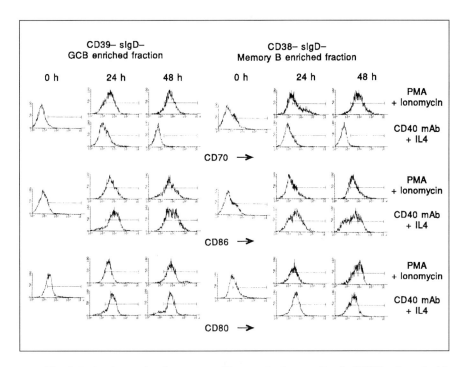

Fig. 8. Activation molecules expressed by germinal center B cells (GCB) cultured with phorbol myristate acetate plus ionomycin or CD40 mAb plus IL-4. FACScan histograms showing phenotypic changes in germinal center B cells and memory B cells after 24 and 48 h culture with either phorbol myristate acetate (PMA) plus ionomycin or CD40 mAb with IL-4. The negative and positive thresholds were set using an irrelevant isotype-matching antibody as the point where 95% of the negative control cells were negative.

nal center and memory B cells treated with CD40 mAb plus IL-4 diverge, those of the same populations treated with phorbol myristate acetate plus ionomycin become markedly similar. Stimulation of germinal center B cells with phorbol myristate acetate plus ionomycin for 24–48 h results in the cells becoming CD44high, CD77low, CD25+, sIghigh, and remaining CD38high and CD23–. This is the phenotype of freshly isolated memory B cells except for the expression of CD38 and CD25, but memory B cells start to express these molecules after treatment with phorbol myristate acetate plus ionomycin.

The phenotype acquired by germinal center B cells on culture with phorbol myristate acetate plus ionomycin is similar to that acquired when they are cocultured with autologous preactivated memory T cells; this suggests that some of the signals these T cells deliver act through protein kinase C.

Conclusion

FDC provide the most obvious source of antigen that must be available if there is to be continued cognate interaction between T and B cells. It is not surprising, therefore, that germinal centers turn out to play an important role in the development of T as well as B cell memory and are probably important in the production of T effector cells as well as plasma cells producing high-affinity antibody. Although germinal centers have been considered for some years to be the domain of immunologists interested in B cells, it is likely that increasingly they will be seen to be central to the study of the response of CD4+ T cells to antigen.

Acknowledgement

Dr. Casamayor-Palleja is supported by an MRC programme grant.

References

1   Kroese FGM, Wubenna AS, Seijen HG, Nieuiwenhuis P: Germinal centers develop oligoclonally. Eur J Immunol 1987;17:1069–1072.
2   Liu Y-J, Zhang J, Lane PJL, Chan EY-T, MacLennan ICM: Sites of specific B cell activation in primary and secondary responses to T cell-dependent and T cell-independent antigens. Eur J Immunol 1991;21:2951–2962.
3   Jacob J, Kelsoe G, Rajewsky K, Weiss U: Intraclonal generation of antibody mutants in germinal centres. Nature 1991;354:389–392.
4   Tew JG, DiLosa RM, Burton GF, Kosco MH, Kupp LI, Masuda A, Szakal AK: Germinal centres and antibody production in bone marrow. Immunol Rev 1992;126:99–112.
5   Smith KGC, Hewitson TD, Nossal GJV, Tarlinton DM: The phenotype and fate of antibody forming cells of the splenic foci. Eur J Immunol 1996;26:444–448.
6   Coico RF, Bhogal BS, Thorbecke GJ: The relationship of germinal centres in lymphoid tissue to immunologic memory. IV. Transfer of B cell memory with lymph node cells fractionated according to their receptors for peanut agglutinin. J Immunol 1983;131:2254–2257.
7   Casamayor-Palleja M, Feuillard J, Ball J, Drew M, MacLennan ICM: Centrocytes rapidly adopt a memory B cell phenotype on co-culture with autologous germinal centre T cell enriched preparations. Int Immunol 1996;8:737–744.
8   Brown JC, Harris G, Papamichail M, Slijivic VS, Holborow EJ: Localization of aggregated human gamma-globulin in the spleens of normal mice. Immunology 1973;24:955–968.
9   Szakal AK, Kosco MH, Tew JG: Microanatomy of lymphoid tissue during the induction and maintenance of humoral immune responses: Structure, function, relationships. Annu Rev Immunol 1989;7:91–111.
10 Zheng B, Xue W, Kelsoe G: Locus specific somatic hypermutation in germinal center T cells. Nature 1994;372:556–559.
11 Gulbranson-Judge A, MacLennan ICM: Sequential antigen-specific growth of T cells in the T zones and follicles in response to pigeon cytochrome c. Eur J Immunol, in press.
12 MacLennan ICM: Germinal centres. Annu Rev Immunol 1994;12:117–139.
13 Jacob J, Kelsoe G: In situ studies of the primary immune response to (4-hydroxy-3-nitrophenyl)acetyl. II. A common clonal origin for periarteriolar lymphoid sheath-associated foci and germinal centres. J Exp Med 1992;176:679–688.

14   Ho F, Lortan J, Khan M, MacLennan ICM: Distinct short-lived and long-lived antibody-producing cell populations. Eur J Immunol 1986;16:1297–1301.

15   Hanna MG: An autoradiographic study of the germinal centre in spleen white pulp during early intervals of the immune response. Lab Invest 1964;13:95–104.

16   Fliedner TM: On the origin of tingible bodies in germinal centres in immune responses; in Cottier H (ed): Germinal Centres in Immune Responses. Berlin, Springer, 1967, pp 218–224.

17   Hardie DL, Johnson GD, Khan M, MacLennan ICM: Quantitative analysis of molecules which distinguish functional compartments within germinal centres. Eur J Immunol 1993;23:997–1004.

18   MacLennan ICM, Gray D: Antigen-driven selection of virgin and memory B cells. Immunol Rev 1986;91:61–85.

19   Liu Y-J, Joshua DE, Williams GT, Smith CA, Gordon J, MacLennan ICM: Mechanisms of antigen driven selection in germinal centre. Nature 1989;342:929–931.

20   Armitage RJ, Fanslow WC, Strockbine L, Sato TA, Clifford KN, MacDuff BM, Anderson DM, Gimple SD, Davis-Smith T, Maliszewiski CR, Clarke EA, Smith CA, Grabstein KH, Cosman D, Spriggs MK: Molecular and biological characterisation of a murine ligand for CD40. Nature 1992; 357:80–82.

21   Lane P, Traunecker A, Hubele S, Inui S, Lanzavecchia A, Gray D: Activated human T cells express a ligand for the human B cell associated antigen CD40 which participates in T cell dependent activation of lymphocytes B. Eur J Immunol 1992;22:2573–2578.

22   Graf D, Korthauer U, Mages HW, Senger G, Kroczek RA: Cloning of TRAP, a ligand for CD40 on human T cells. Eur J Immunol 1992;22:3191–3194.

23   Lederman S, Yellin M, Inghirami G, Lee J, Knowles D, Chess L: Molecular interactions mediating T-B lymphocyte collaboration in human lymphoid follicles: Roles of T cell-B cell activating molecule (5c8 antigen) and CD40 in contact-dependent help. J Immunol 1992;149:3817–3826.

24   Holder MJ, Wang H, Milner AE, Casamayor M, Armitage R, Spriggs MK, Fanslow WC, MacLennan ICM, Gregory CD, Gordon J: Suppression of apoptosis in normal and neoplastic human B lymphocytes by CD40 ligand is independent of bcl-2 induction. Eur J Immunol 1993;23:2368–2371.

25   Lagresle C, Bella C, Defrance T: Phenotype and functional heterogeneity of the IgD-B cell compartment: Identification of two major tonsillar B cell subsets. Int Immunol 1993;5:1259–1268.

26   Pascual V, Liu YJ, Maglaski A, de Bouteiller O, Bancherau J, Capra JD: Analysis of somatic mutation in five B cell subsets in human tonsil. J Exp Med 1994;180:329–339.

27   Liu Y-J, Barthelemy C, de Bouteiller O, Arpin C, Durand I, Bancherau J: Memory B cells from human tonsils colonize mucosal epithelium and directly present antigen to T cells by rapid upregulation of B7.1 and B7.2. Immunity 1995;2:239–248.

28   Feuillard J, Taylor D, Casamayor-Palleja M, Johnson GD, MacLennan ICM: Isolation and characteristics of tonsil centroblasts with reference to Ig class switching. Int Immunol 1995;7:121–130.

29   Lagresle C, Bella C, Daniel PT, Krammer PH, Defrance T: Regulation of germinal center B cell differentiation. Role of the human APO-1/Fas (CD95) molecule. J Immunol 1995;154:5746–5756.

30   Mangeney M, Rousselet G, Taga S, Tursz T, Wiels J: The fate of human CD77+ germinal center B lymphocytes after rescue from apoptosis. Mol Immunol 1995;5:333–339.

31   Arpin C, Dechanet J, van Kooten C, Merville P, Grouard G, Brière F, Bancherau J, Liu YJ: Generation of memory and plasma cells in vitro. Science 1995;5211:720–722.

32   Chan EYT, MacLennan ICM: Only a small proportion of splenic B-cells in adults are short-lived virgin cells. Eur J Immunol 1993;23:357–363.

33   Casamayor-Palleja M, Khan M, MacLennan ICM: A subset of CD4+ memory T cells contains preformed CD40 ligand that is rapidly but transiently expressed on their surface after activation through the T cell receptor. J Exp Med 1995;181:1293–1301.

34   Yellin MJ, Sippel K, Inghirami G, Covey LR, Lee JJ, Sinning J, Clark EA, Chess L, Lederman S: CD40 molecules induce down-regulation and endocytosis of T cell surface T cell-B cell activating molecule/CD40L. Potential role in regulating helper effector function. J Immunol 1994;152:598–608.

35   Akbar AN, Terry L, Timms A, Beverley PCL, Janossy G: Loss of CD45R and gain of UCHL 1 reactivity is a feature of primed T cells. J Immunol 1988;140:2171–2178.

36   Kelsoe G, Zheng B: Sites of B-cell activation in vivo. Curr Opin Immunol 1993;5:418–422.
37   Fuller KA, Kanagawa O, Nahm MH: T cells within germinal centres are specific for the immunizing antigen. J Immunol 1993;151:4505–4512.
38   Vaux DL, Cory S, Adams JM: Bcl-2 gene promotes hematopoietic-cell survival and cooperates with c-Myc to immortalize pre-B cells. Nature 1988;335:440–442.
39   Kepler TB, Perelson AS: Cyclic reentry of germinal centre B-cells and the efficiency of affinity maturation. Immunol Today 1993;14:412–415.
40   Han SH, Hathcock K, Zheng B, Kepler TB, Hodes R, Kelsoe G: Cellular interaction in germinal centres. Roles of CD40 ligand and B7-1 and B7-2 in established germinal centres. J Immunol 1995; 155:556–567.
41   Grammer AC, Bergman MC, Miura Y, Fugita K, Davis LS, Lipsky PE: The CD40 ligand expressed by human B cells costimulates B-cell responses. J Immunol 1995;154:4996–5010.
42   Brachtel EF, Washiyama M, Johnson GD, Tenner-Racz K, Racz P, MacLennan ICM: Differences in the germinal centres of palatine tonsils and lymph nodes. Scand J Immunol 1996;43:239–247.
43   Küppers R, Zhao-Hohn M, Hansmann M, Rajewsky K: Tracing B cell development in human germinal centres by molecular analysis of single cells picked from histological sections. EMBO J 1993;12:4955–4967.
44   Martinez-Valdez H, Guret C, Deboutellier O, Fugier I, Banchereau J, Liu Y-J: Human germinal center B cells express the apoptosis inducing genes Fas, c-myc, p-53, and Bax but not the survival gene Bcl-2. J Exp Med 1996;183:971–977.
45   Andersson E, Ohlin M, Borrebaeck CAK, Carlsson R: CD4(+) CD57(+) T cells derived from peripheral-blood do not support immunoglobulin production by B cells. Cell Immunol 1995;163: 245–253.
46   Bouzahzah F, Bosseloir A, Heinen E, Simar LI: Human germinal centre CD4(+) CD57(+) T cells act differently on B cells than do classical T helper cells. Dev Immunol 1995;4:189–197.
47   Prince HE, York J, Jensen ER: Phenotypic comparison of the three populations of human lymphocytes defined by CD45RO and CD45RA expression. Cell Immunol 1992;145:245–262.
48   Parra E, Wingren AG, Sjogren H-O, Kalland T, Sansom D, Dohlsten M: Human naive and memory T helper cells display distinct adhesion properties to ICAM-1, LFA 3 and B7 molecules. Scand J Immunol 1993;38:508–514.
49   MacLennan ICM: Mechanisms of B Cell Neoplasia. Session II: B cells. Basel, Roche, 1989, p 103–182.
50   Ren CL, Ru SM, Geha RS: Protein tyrosine kinase C translocation are functional components of CD40 signal transduction in resting B cells. Immunol Invest 1994;23:437–448.
51   Marshall LS, Sheperd DM, Ledbetter JA, Aruffo A, Noelle RJ: Signalling events during helper T cell dependent B cell activation. 1. Analysis of the signal transduction pathways triggered by activated helper T cell in resting B cells. J Immunol 1994;152:4816–4825.
52   Kato T, Kokuho T, Tamura T, Nariuchi H: Mechanisms of T cell contact dependent B cell activation. J Immunol 1994;152:2130–2138.
53   Lalmanach-Girard AC, Chiles TC, Parker DC, Rothstein TL: T cell dependent induction of NF-kappa-B in B cells. J Exp Med 1993;177:1215–1219.
54   Huo L, Rothstein TL: Receptor specific induction of individual AP-1 components in B lymphocytes. J Immunol 1995;154:3300–3309.

Prof. I.C.M. MacLennan, Department of Immunology,
University of Birmingham Medical School, Birmingham B15 2TT (UK)

Ferrarini M, Caligaris-Cappio F (eds): Human B Cell Populations.
Chem Immunol. Basel, Karger, 1997, vol 67, pp 45–57

....

Biased VH4 Gene Segment Repertoire in the Human Tonsil

Virginia Pascual[a], Patrick Wilson[a], Yong-Jun Liu[b], Jacques Banchereau[c], J. Donald Capra[a]

[a] Department of Microbiology, University of Texas Southwestern Medical Center, Dallas, Tex., USA;
[b] Schering-Plough Laboratory for Immunological Research, Dardilly, France;
[c] Baylor Institute for Immunological Research, Dallas, Tex., USA

The variable regions of the two critical antigen receptors of the immune system, the T cell receptor and the immunoglobulin molecule (Ig), are encoded by five different genetic elements that in the germline are separated by many thousands of base pairs [1, 2]. A recombination machinery brings these elements together into functional TCR Vβ/Vα and Ig VH/VL chains [3]. Availability of a wide array of germline genes, generation of random amino acids during the process of rearrangement, and combinatorial association of variable region chains are essential steps in the generation of diversity within the T and B repertoires. B cells display the unique property of being able to accumulate somatic mutations within their Ig variable region genes, further contributing to expand the already broad array of antigenic specificities [1]. A subset of murine germinal center T cells has been recently reported to display somatic mutations at the Vα gene level, but the relevance of this phenomenon in humans is yet unknown [4].

Peripheral lymphoid organs provide the microenvironment for the activation of virgin and memory B cells and the accumulation of somatic mutations during the humoral immune response. Early B cell activation during antigen-specific antibody responses occurs in the T cell and interdigitating cell areas of the lymph nodes, tonsils, Peyer patches, and the periarteriolar lymphocytic sheaths of the spleen. This early B cell activation gives rise to short-lived plasma cells, IgM (+) splenic marginal zone B cells, and primary B cell blasts that colonize the primary follicles [5–8]. The subsequent germinal center reaction (GC) is initiated by the rapid proliferation of three to five primary blasts in association with follicular dendritic cells [5, 6, 9]. The primary B cell blast follows a differentiation pathway from centroblast to centrocyte, and then to either a plasma or a memory B cell [10–13]. During these processes, somatic hypermutation [14–17], positive selection [18–20], and differentiation of high affinity GC B cells take place [18–26].

Liu et al. [27] recently described the separation of human tonsillar B cells into fractions representing different stages of B cell differentiation. Using of a series of phenotypic markers that include sIgD, sIgM, sIgG, CD23, CD44, Bcl-2, CD38, CD10, CD77, and Ki67, pure populations of follicular mantle (Bm1 and Bm2), germinal center (Bm3 and Bm4), and memory B cells (Bm5) were obtained (fig. 1). To establish whether the initiation of somatic mutation correlates with this phenotypic characterization, we performed polymerase chain reaction (PCR) and subsequent sequencing analysis of the Ig heavy chain variable region genes from each of the B cell subsets. In agreement with previous reports, we found that the somatic mutation machinery is activated only after B cells reach the GC and become centroblasts (Bm3). Whereas 47 independently rearranged IgM transcripts from the Bm1 and Bm2 subsets were nearly germline-encoded, 57 Bm3-Bm5 transcripts had accumulated an average of 5.7 point mutations within the VH gene segment. Gamma transcripts corresponding to the same VH gene families were isolated from subsets Bm3, Bm4, and Bm5, and had accumulated an average of 9.5 point mutations. These findings confirm that the molecular events underlying the process of somatic mutation take place during the transition from IgD+, CD23+ B cell (Bm2) to the IgD–, CD23– GC centroblast (Bm3). Furthermore, the analysis of Ig variable region gene transcripts from the different B cell subpopulations confirmed that the pathway of B cell differentiation from the virgin or naive stage, through the GC, up to the memory compartment could be traced with phenotypic markers [28]

The human VH locus contains approximately 100 different genes, 50% of which are pseudogenes [29, 30]. Only a few out of the 50 functional VH gene segments, however, are recurrently found when bulk peripheral blood B cells are studied [31–34]. One of the most frequently found VH genes, VH4-21, has been the subject of extensive analysis in our laboratory [34]. The VH4-21 (VH4.34) gene segment encodes most human cold agglutinins as well as a broad array of different autospecificities like RF and anti-DNA. In fact, serological analyses using the anti-idiotypic antibody 9G4 which recognizes the product of the VH4-21 gene segment showed that Ig expressing this VH gene segment are overrepresented in patients with SLE, especially during the active phases of the disease [35]. The same anti-idiotypic antibody (9G4) originally described by Stevenson et al. [36] was used to analyze fetal spleen and normal adult peripheral blood and lymphoid tissues with striking results. These authors showed that the percentage of idiotype-positive cells ranged from 10.9% in the normal adult bone marrow to 6.9% in the peripheral blood, down to 2.9% in total tonsil B cells. In contrast, less than 1% of the pool of circulating IgM and IgG proteins expressed the idiotypic

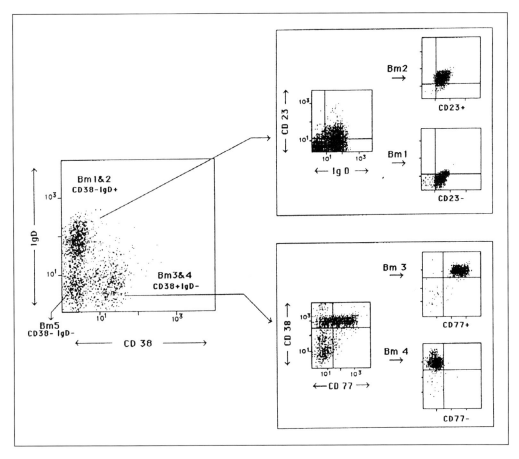

Fig. 1. Immunofluorescence FACS analysis of tonsil B cells to identify IgD+ CD38–
FM B cells, IgD– CD38+ GC B cells, and IgD– CD38– memory B cells. IgD+ cells are
further sorted into CD23– (Bm1) and CD23+ (Bm2). CD38+ cells are sorted into CD77+
(Bm3), and CD77– (Bm4) cells.

marker. Our group recently established that the VH4-21-specific idiotope responsible for the interaction with the 9G4 antibody is located at the 3′ end of the first
framework region [37]. Because this region is usually well preserved even in highly mutated VH4-21-encoded antibodies, the results of the idiotypic analysis suggest that counterselection rather than somatic mutation within the B cells expressing this gene segment is the main mechanism responsible for the progressive loss
of idiotype expression throughout B cell differentiation, especially at the level of
secreted protein. As described previously, VH4-21 overexpression within mature

B cells is in sharp contrast with the scarce amount of secreted VH4-21-encoded protein in normal human sera, suggesting that B cells expressing the product of the VH4-21 gene segment may be the subject of immune selection at some point during B cell differentiation, most likely around the transition from germinal center to plasma cells.

VH4-21-encoded antibodies also bind to CD45, a membrane glycoprotein expressed on most human B lymphocytes and structurally related to the i antigen, one of the targets of the cold agglutinin response [38]. The interaction between VH4-21-encoded antibodies and B cells has been reported to result in biological effects in vitro, including cytotoxicity. Interestingly, VH4-21-mediated cytotoxicity seems to be independent of apoptosis or complement fixation but mediated through the formation of cell membrane pores that can be visualized by scanning electron microscopy [39].

Apart from its interesting binding capacities, the product of the VH4-21 gene segment displays a rather remarkable pattern of expression among human lymphoid malignancies, the most striking being its overwhelming representation within large-cell diffuse lymphoma, a tumor of germinal center origin, together with a complete absence from the repertoire of human myelomas that derive from plasma cells within the bone marrow [40, 41]. This pattern of expression suggests that selection of the Ig VH repertoire is regulated through the different compartments of B cell differentiation, a hypothesis that we have tested using tonsillar B cell subpopulations in the experiments that we will describe below.

Materials and Methods

Isolation of Tonsil B Cells
Tonsil samples were taken during tonsillectomy. The samples were minced, and the resulting cell suspensions subjected to two rounds of T cell depletion using 2-aminoethylisothioridium bromide-modified sheep red blood cells. The resulting cells were further separated into high density and low density B cells by centrifugation through 15, 60, and 65% Percoll gradients. These cells were used for phenotypic analysis, immunomagnetic bead sorting, and FACS sorting, as described [27]. To isolate plasma cells, total tonsillar cell suspensions were obtained by pulling apart tonsils with tweezers and digesting the remaining tissue twice with 1 mg/ml collagenase and 0.1 U/ml DNAse in RPMI 1640 at 37°C for 20 min. To remove small cells and enrich for plasma cells, cellular suspensions were centrifuged 3 or 4 times (10 g, 20 min, 4°C) on PBS 1.5% BSA. Plasma cells were then labeled at 4°C with PE-conjugated anti-CD38 mAb either alone or in combination with FITC-conjugated anti-CD20 mAb, and sorted at 4°C.

Sequencing the Ig VH/VL Transcripts from the Different B Cell Subpopulations
Total RNA was extracted using guanidinium thiocyanate-phenol-chloroform in a single step [42] and reverse-transcribed using oligo d(T) as primer and avian myeloblastosis virus reverse transcriptase. First strand cDNA was directly used for second strand synthesis

---

and amplification via PCR using primers corresponding to the Cμ, and Cγ constant regions in combination with the VH4, VH5, and VH6 family-specific leader oligonucleotides, as described [28, 43]. The PCR products were purified using microconcentrators, kinased, and blunt-end-ligated into an EcoRV-digested, dephosphorylated plasmid, as previously described. After transformation and screening with consensus internal oligonucleotides, positive colonies were picked up and the plasmids were sequenced using fluorescent-labelled ddNTP and Taq polymerase in an automated sequencer. The resulting sequences were compared to the germline using DNAstar (DNAstar, Madison, Wisc., USA).

Immunostaining Analysis

Portions of tonsils were snap-frozen in liquid nitrogen and stored at −70°C. Five-micrometer frozen sections were cut and mounted on glass slides, dried at room temperature for 1 h and fixed in acetone at 4°C for 15 min. Sections were stained by double immunoenzyme technique using the biotin-avidin-peroxidase system and the alkaline phosphatase anti-alkaline phosphatase system, as described [27]. 9G4 and LC1 mAbs were kindly provided by Dr. Stevenson and Dr. Jefferis, respectively.

Results

The VH4-21 Gene Segment Encodes the Majority of VH4 Gene Products in the IgM-Expressing B Cell Subpopulations of the Human Tonsil

We have generated VH4-specific Ig gene libraries using RNA from each of the tonsil subpopulations of two normal donors. The libraries were constructed using different constant region-specific oligonucleotides to subclone all possible VH4-expressing isotypes. Replica filter screening with VH4-21-specific oligonucleotides corresponding to conserved regions of this gene, as well as with constant region probes to detect double positives, disclosed a progressive decrease in the frequency of VH4-21 transcripts as B cell differentiation progressed from the IgM to the IgG compartment (fig. 2). Sequence analyses of over 150 transcripts from each of the subpopulations confirmed the screening results and are summarized below. Basically, the overrepresentation of the VH4-21 gene segment is strikingly maintained during the transition of follicular mantle B cells into the IgM-expressing population of centroblasts and centrocytes in the GC up to the IgM memory compartment, to decline significantly in cells that express gamma isotype. These results suggest that, regardless of the B cell differentiation stage, some of the selective events responsible for shaping the Ig repertoire in the periphery take place around the time of isotype switching.

By performing centrifugation of total tonsil suspensions over 1.5% BSA at 10 g, Merville et al. [44] have recently been able to enrich tonsillar plasma cells from an initial 1–2% to about 8% of the total tonsillar cells. Subsequent sorting according to CD38 and CD20 expression allows the isolation of 90% pure plasma cells displaying typical morphological and ultrastructural characteristics. Our

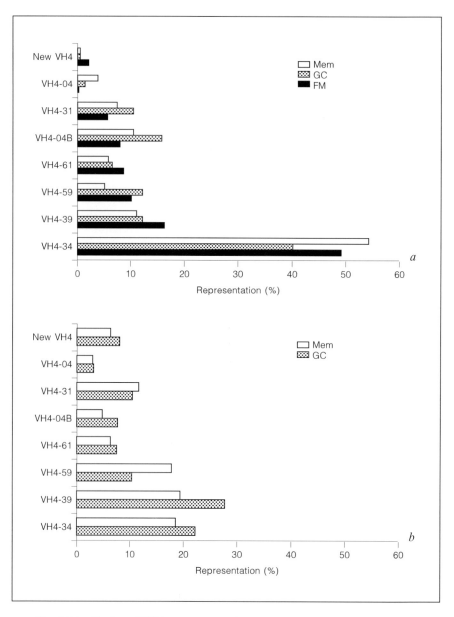

Fig. 2. Distribution of VH4 gene segments in FM, GC, and memory (Mem) IgM transcripts of the tonsil (*a*) and GC and memory IgG transcripts (*b*).

analysis of the human plasma cell VH4 repertoire within the human tonsil is summarized in figure 2. Interestingly, the percentage of VH4-21 (+) transcripts decreased from 50% in GC cells to 10% in the IgM-secreting plasma cell compartment. The frequency of VH4-21-encoded transcripts did not change significantly, however, in the transition from GC to IgG-secreting plasma cells.

VH4 is the most homogeneous human VH family, the majority of VH4 gene segments sharing almost identical nucleotide sequence throughout the FW regions while displaying only a few differences in CDR1 and CDR2. The VH4-21 gene segment, however, is the most distant member of this family, exhibiting 95% identity at the nucleotide level with the consensus VH4 sequence. Some of these nucleotide differences lead to unique amino acid substitutions at the 3′ end of the FW1 region and give rise to an idiotypic determinant that is recognized by the rat mAb 9G4. The structural basis of this idiotype has been extensively characterized in our laboratory. The idiotype is present in the vast majority of VH4-21-encoded antibodies tested to date, and is responsible for the cross-reactivity observed many years ago when human cold agglutinins were tested against rabbit anti-idiotypic antisera [45]. More recently, it was noticed that antibodies encoded by VH4 family members other than VH4-21 share a different idiotypic determinant recognized by the LC1 mAb [46, 47]. Once again, Potter et al. [37] in our laboratory studied the structural basis of this idiotype and found that it mapped to the same FW1 region where VH4-21 and 9G4 interact. Mabs 9G4 and LC1 therefore provide us with excellent tools to analyze the expression of the VH4-21 gene segment and compare it with all the other members of the family in staining experiments. The results of these experiments confirm the sequencing data described above. Most FM regions in 8 tonsils analyzed to date contain VH4-expressing B cells, of which around 50% are consistently VH4-21 (+). The most striking observation derived from these studies, however, is the paucity of GC immune complexes containing VH4-21 encoded IgG (1–5%), as opposed to other VH4 family members that range from 16 to 30% of the total content of GC immune complexes, as detected by the LC1 mAb [data not shown]. These data again support the notion that while VH4-21/IgM-expressing B cells are not only allowed but overrepresented in the primary repertoire, some selective mechanism censors their successful differentiation into fully secreting plasma cells.

Sequence Analyses Reveal that Somatic Diversification in the Human GC Is Not Restricted to Point Mutation

We have reported that a correlation exists between germinal center B cell phenotype and initiation of somatic mutation within VH genes. Additionally, we confirmed the notion previously described by several other groups of mutational preference/strand polarity, i.e. a bias towards favoring the mutation of particular nucleotides as well as one of the two DNA strands [28]. In our recent extensive analyses of VH4 transcripts from Bm1-Bm5 populations, we have found additional mutational events that have not been reported previously in the human, in particular the insertion/deletion of codons within hypervariable regions (data not shown). Codon insertion/deletion are rare events (they involve 1–2% of the transcripts) and display several very interesting characteristics. They are exclusively seen within CDRs, resembling the diversification mechanism used to generate germline VH4 family genes, which are very homologous at the nucleotide level but exhibit different CDR1 lengths. Additionally, they exclusively involve GC and memory B cells, the two subsets that constitute the target and result of somatic mutation, respectively.

In order to gain additional insight into the relevance and frequency of these observations, it was important to definitively prove the absence of a germline counterpart for what we believe is a somatic process. We, therefore, needed to rule out the existence of allelic variants within the germline of the donor containing the putative sequence variants. The analysis of over 1,000 VH4 transcripts from 2 independent tonsils firmly supports the somatic nature of these phenomena. While in one of the donors it was relatively easy to identify a novel member/allele of the VH4 family based on its recurrent appearance in different subpopulations, including FM cells expressing unmutated sequences, none of the insertion/deletion events was found more than once in the same form or within identical CDRs, suggesting again that they are not germline-imprinted. Additionally, cloning and sequencing the germline members of the VH4 family from one of the donor's DNA failed to disclose any of the variants found within the GC/memory compartments.

Discussion

Most of our current knowledge concerning the generation of human antibody specificities has been either extrapolated from the murine system or based on an analysis of the products of immortalized B cells. Furthermore, the phenotypic characterization of the B cells involved in normal and autoimmune antibody responses has not been fully elucidated. Many controversial reports exist for example regarding the contribution of specific B cell subsets, like the B1 or CD5+ cells, to autoimmunity [48]. The controversy is somewhat sustained by the artificial modulation of the expression of some B cell phenotypic markers during the various processes of immortalization. Although a large body of information regarding antibody variable region gene usage in autoimmune responses has accumulated in recent years, the relevance of the structural data may be questioned if not placed in the context of the differentiation stage of the cells assembling and expressing these antibodies. It is well known for example that the normal bone marrow and peripheral blood B cell repertoires express specificities against self [49, 50]. Under normal circumstances, however, self-reactive cells do not expand and secrete their immunoglobulin gene products. A constellation of factors involving each of the sequential steps that participate in the selection and activation of B cells, both centrally and peripherally, may be responsible for this tolerization. In the mouse, it has been postulated that negative selection in the bone marrow leads to the purging of up to 50% of the B cells with recently assembled Ig receptors due to their germline-imprinted reactivity against self [51]. Peripherally, however, somatic mutation of Ig gene segments not only contributes to diversify the B cell repertoire and generate high affinity antibodies, but may lead also to the reappearance of certain self-specificities. Lack of T cell help, and apoptosis of B cells with decreased affinity toward foreign triggering antigens during the GC reaction are mechanisms likely to contribute to the silencing of self-reactive mutants.

Having access to pure subpopulations of mature peripheral B cells as well as plasma cells, we decided to test the hypothesis of whether repertoire selection may be implemented through the various differentiation stages of these cells by analyzing the frequency of VH4-21 gene segment expression compared to other VH4 family members. As figure 2 shows, we found a striking overrepresentation of B cells expressing VH4-21 gene products within the FM, GC, and memory IgM-expressing compartments. This frequency, however, decreases by half upon switching to IgG. The observation that switching from the μ to the γ isotype correlates best with changes in VH4-21 gene segment expression suggests that the binding pattern and/or the epitopes responsible for selection of the antibody molecule may be influenced not only by the variable region, but also by the combination of variable and constant regions.

Somatic hypermutation is one of the major mechanisms contributing to the diversification of the Ig repertoire. It is a B cell-specific process that takes place preferentially within germinal centers in peripheral lymphoid organs. To date, very little is known about the signals triggering mutation and the cellular machinery responsible for its implementation. Although in the human base pair exchange is considered to be the major mutational event, other species like the chicken, the rabbit, or the sheep use different mechanisms like gene conversion to cover their repertoire needs [52–54]. The process of somatic hypermutation targets exlusively the DNA within and around rearranged Ig variable region genes, from the upstream leader intron to the 3′ JH intronic area, spanning a total of approximately 1.5 kb of DNA [55]. However, transgenic models in which non-Ig genes are designed to replace the coding variable region also accumulate mutations, suggesting that the targeted sequence itself is not responsible for triggering the mutation process [56]. Additionally, it has recently been reported that somatic mutation is linked to the initiation of transcription: when an extra Ig promoter is artificially placed upstream of the light chain constant region, both the VJ and the C regions, but not the intervening sequences, mutate at similar rates [57].

An interesting observation derived from our analyses of hundreds of VH transcript sequences from each of the tonsillar subpopulations is the occasional finding of amino acid insertion/deletion phenomena within the antibody variable region. These events are found at low frequency, and are exclusively restricted to the IgG expressing GC and memory compartments of the human tonsil, supporting their somatic origin. Furthermore, we have detected them within the hypervariable regions or CDRs, an observation that may be explained by the fact that these regions encode loops with less structural length constraints than the frameworks. Additionally, all the insertion/deletion events involve full codons, as expected by the fact that the cells that we analyzed had been selected with phenotypic markers, some of which include sIg, and are consequently expected to express functional Ig molecules.

Insertion/deletion mismatches (IDL) are considered one of the germline DNA damage mechanisms that are the target of the repair machinery in higher eukaryotic cells. A failure of the cell to recognize and repair such damage is a key early step in tumor progression. Under normal circumstances, DNA damage leads to an increase in activity of p53 with the subsequent activation of p21/WAF1, GADD45, and mdm2, leading to growth arrest or apoptosis. In a recent report, Lee et al. [58] described the specific binding of p53 and its 14-kDa C-terminal domain to DNAs containing 1–3 IDL mismatches. While only background binding was observed by electron microscopy to the site of a G/T mismatch, strong binding to a 3-base bulge, and even stronger to three closely spaced bulges was noticed. Interestingly, gel retardation studies revealed p53-DNA complexes around IDL mismatches to be highly stable (half-life of >2 h), suggesting that upon encountering these lesions, p53 may recruit other proteins to the damaged site. In summary, even though GC B cells are the only known target for the generation of physiologically regulated DNA mutations, very little is currently known about the DNA repair mechanisms within these cells, and it is indeed possible that both conventional DNA repair enzymes as well as a novel, yet to be described mismatch/repair and/or polymerase enzymes with low proof-reading capacity are involved in the generation of GC somatic mutants. Experiments are currently underway to address some of these interesting issues.

References

1   Tonegawa S: Somatic generation of antibody diversity. Nature 1983;302:575.
2   Kronenberg M, Siu G, Hood LE, Shasstri N: The molecular genetics of the T cell antigen receptor and T-cell antigen recognition. Annu Rev Immunol 1986;4:529.
3   Schatz DG, Baltimore D: Stable expression of immunoglobulin gene V(D)J recombinase activity by gene transfer into 3T3 fibroblasts. Cell 1988;53:107.
4   Zheng B, Xue W, Kelsoe G: Locus-specific somatic hypermutation in germinal center T cells. Nature 1994;372:556.
5   Liu Y-J, Zhang J, Lane PJL, Chan Y-T, MacLennan ICM: Sites of specific B cell activation in primary and secondary responses to T cell-dependent and T cell-independent antigens. Eur J Immunol 1991;21:2951.
6   Jacob J, Kassir R, Kelsoe G: In situ studies of the primary immune response to (4-hydroxy-3-nitrophenyl) acetyl. I. The architecture and dynamics of responding cell populations. J Exp Med 1991;173:1165.
7   Claassen E, Kors E, Dijkstra CD, Van Rooijen N: Marginal zone of the spleen and the development and localization of specific antibody forming cells against thymus-dependent and thymus-independent type-2 antigens. Immunology 1986;57:399.
8   Liu Y-J, Oldfield S, MacLennan ICM: Memory B cells in T cell-dependent antibody responses colonize the splenic marginal zones. Eur J Immunol 1988;18:355.
9   Kroese FGM, Wubbena AS, Seijen HG, Nieuwenhuis P: Germinal centers develop oligoclonally. Eur J Immunol 1987;17:1069.
10 Liu Y-J, Johnson GD, Gordon J, MacLennan ICM: Germinal centers in T cell-dependent antibody responses. Immunol Today 1992;13:17.
11 MacLennan J, Liu Y-J, Johnson GD: Maturation and dispersal of B-cell clones during T cell-dependent antibody responses. Immunol Rev 1992;126:143.
12 Jacob J, Kelsoe G, Rajewsky K, Weiss U: Intraclonal generation of antibody mutants in germinal centers. Nature 1990;354:389.
13 Weiss U, Rajewsky K: The repertoire of somatic antibody mutants accumulating in the memory compartment after primary immunization restricted through affinity maturation and mirrors that expressed in the secondary response. J Exp Med 1990;172:1681.
14 Berek C, Berger A, Apel M: Maturation of the immune response in germinal centers. Cell 1991;67: 1121.
15 Leanderson T, Kallberg E, Gray D: Expansion, selection and mutation of antigen-specific B cells in germinal centers. Immunol Rev 1992;126:47.
16 Liu Y-J, Joshua DA, Williams GT, Smith CA, Gordon J, MacLennan ICM: Mechanism of antigen-driven selection in germinal centers. Nature 1989;342:929.
17 Liu Y-J, Mason DY, Johnson GD, Abbot S, Gregory GD, Hardie DL, Gordon J, MacLennan ICM: Germinal center cells express bcl-2 protein after activation by signals which prevent their entry into apoptosis. Eur J Immunol 1991;21:1905.
18 Foote J, Milstein C: Kinetic maturation of an immune response. Nature 1991;353:530.
19 Klaus GGB, Humphrey JH, Kunkel A, Dongworth DW: The follicular dendritic cell: Its role in antigen presentation in the generation of immunological memory. Immunol Rev 1990;53:3.
20 Coico RF, Bhogal BS, Thorbecke GJ: Relationship of germinal centers in lymphoid tissue to immunologic memory. IV. Transfer of B cell memory with lymph node cells fractionated according to their receptors for peanut agglutinin. J Immunol 1983;131:2254.
21 Tsiagbe VK, Linton P-J, Thorbecke GJ: The path of memory B-cell development. Immunol Rev 1992;126:113.
22 Kosco MH, Burton GF, Kapasi ZF, Szakal AK, Tew JG: Antibody-forming cell induction during an early phase of germinal center development and its delay with ageing. Immunology 1989;68:312.
23 Tew JG, DiLosa R-M, Burton GF, Kosco MH, Kupp LI, Masuda A, Szakal AK: Germinal centers and antibody production in bone marrow. Immunol Rev 1992;126:99.

24   Liu Y-J, Cairns JA, Holder MJ, Abbot SD, Jansen KU, Bonnefoi JY, Gordon J, MacLennan ICM: Recombinant 25-kDa CD23 and interleukin 1a promote the survival of germinal center B cells: Evidence for the bifurcation in the development of centrocytes rescued from apoptosis. Eur J Immunol 1991;21:1107.

25   McLennan ICM: The center of hypermutation. Nature 1991;354:352.

26   Nossal GJV: The molecular and cellular basis of affinity maturation in the antibody response. Cell 1992;68:1.

27   Liu Y-J, de Bouteiller O, Arpin C, Durand I, Banchereau J: Five human mature B cell subsets; in Heinen E, Defresne MP, Boniver J, Geenen V (eds): In vivo Immunology. New York, Plenum Press, 1994, pp 289–294.

28   Pascual V, Liu Y-J, Magalski A, Banchereau J, Capra JD: Analysis of somatic mutation in five B cell subsets. J Exp Med 1994;180:329.

29   Matsuda F, Shin EK, Nagaoka H, Matsumura R, Haino M, Fukita Y, Taka-ishi S, Imai T, Riley JH, Anand R, Soeda E, Honjo T: Structure and physical map of 64 variable segments in the 3′ 0.8-megabase region of the human immunoglobulin heavy chain locus. Nature Genet 1993;3:88–94.

30   Cook GH, Tomlinson IM, Walter G, Riethman H, Carter NP, Buluwela L, Winter G, Rabbits TH: A complete map of the human immunoglobulin VH locus on the telomeric region of chromosome 14q. Nature Genet 1994;7:162–168.

31   Kraj P, Friedman DF, Stevenson F, Silberstein LE: Evidence for the overexpression of the VH4-34 (VH4.21) Ig gene segment in the normal adult peripheral blood B cell repertoire. J Immunol 1995; 1545:6406–6420.

32   Suzuki I, Pfister L, Glas A, Nottenburg C, Milner EC: Representation of rearranged VH gene segments in the human adult antibody repertoire. J Immunol 1995;154:3902–3911.

33   Stewart AK, Huang C, Stollar BD, Schwartz RS: High frequency representation of a single VH gene in the expressed human B cell repertoire. J Exp Med 1993;177:409–418.

34   Demaison C, David D, Letourneur F, Theze J, Saragosti S, Zouali M: Analysis of human VH repertoire expression in peripheral CD19(+) B cells. Immunogenetics 1995;42:342–352.

35   Isenberg D, Spellberberg M, Williams M, Griffiths M, Stevenson F: Identification of the 9G4 idiotope in SLE. Br J Rheumatol 1993;32:876.

36   Stevenson FK, Smith GJ, Noerth J, Hamblin TJ, Glennie MJ: Identification of normal B cell counterparts of neoplastic B cells which secrete cold agglutinins of anti-i and anti-I specificity. Br J Haematol 1989;72:9.

37   Potter K, Li Y, Pascual V, Williams R, Spellerberg M, Stevenson F, Capra JD: Molecular characterization of a major cross-reactive idiotype on human immunoglobulins utilizing the VH4-21 gene segment. J Exp Med 1993;178:1419.

38   Grillot-Courvalin C, Brouet JC, Piller F, Rassenti LZ, Labaume S, Silverman GJ, Silberstein LE, Kipps TJ: The anti-B cell autoantibodies from Wiskott-Aldrich syndrome recognizes i blood group specificity on B cells. Eur J Immunol 1992;22:1781.

39   Bhat NM, Bieber MM, Stevenson FK, Teng NNH: Rapid cytotoxicity of human B lymphocytes induced by VH4-34 (VH4-21) gene-encoded monoclonal antibodies. Clin Exp Med, in press.

40   Hsu FJ, Levy R: Preferential use of the VH4 Ig gene family by diffuse large-cell lymphoma. Blood 1995;86:3072–3082.

41   Rettig MB, Vescio RA, Cao J, Wu CH, Lee JC, Han E, DerDanielian M, Newman R, Hong C, Lichtenstein AK, Berenson JR: VH gene usage in multiple myeloma: Complete absence of the VH4-21 (VH4-34) gene. Blood 1995;87:2846–2852.

42   Chomczynski P, Sacchi N: Single step method of RNA isolation by acid guanidinium thiocyanate-phenol-chloroform extraction. Anal Biochem 1987;162:156.

43   Marks JD, Tristem M, Karpas A, Winter G: Oligonucleotide primers for polymerase chain reaction amplification of human immunoglobulin variable genes and design of family-specific oligonucleotide probes. Eur J Immunol 1991;21:985.

44   Merville P, Dechanet J, Desmouliere A, Durand I, de Bouteiller O, Garrone P, Banchereau J, Liu Y-J: BCL-2 (+) tonsillar plasma cells are rescued from apoptosis by bone marrow fibroblasts. J Exp Med 1996;183:227–236.

45   Ono M, Winearls CG, Amos N, Grennan D, Gharavi A, Peters DK, Sissons JGP: Monoclonal antibodies to restricted and cross-reactive idiotopes on monoclonal rheumatoid factors and their recognition of idiotope-positive cells. Eur J Immunol 1987;17:343–349.

46   Pratt LF, Szubin R, Carson DA, Kipps TJ: Molecular characterization of a supratypic cross-reactive idiotype associated with IgM autoantibodies. J Immunol 1991;147:2041–2046.

47   Potter K, Li YC, Capra JD: The cross-reactive idiotopes recognized by the monoclonal antibodies 9G4 and LC1 are located in framework region 1 on two non-overlapping subsets of human VH4 family encoded antibodies. Scand J Immunol 1994;40:43–49.

48   Hardy R, Carmack C, Sheng Y, Hayakawa K: Distinctive developmental origins and specificities of murine CD5+B cells. Immunol Rev 1994;137:91.

49   Kerney J, Vakil M: Idiotype-directed interactions during ontogeny play a major role in the establishment of the adult repertoire. Immunol Rev 1986;94:39.

50   Coutinho A: Beyond clonal selection and network. Immunol Rev 1989;110:264.

51   Deenen G, Van Balen I, Opstelten D: In rat B lymphocyte genesis 60% is lost from the bone marrow at the transition of non-dividing pre-B cell to sIgM+ lymphocyte, the stage of Ig light chain gene expression. Eur J Immunol 1990;20:537.

52   Reynaud CA, Dahan A, Anquez V, Weill JC: Somatic hyperconversion diversifies the single VH gene of the chicken with a high incidence in the D region. Cell 1989;59:171–183.

53   Knight KL, Becker RS: Molecular basis of the allelic inheritance of rabbit immunoglobulin VH allotypes: Implications for the generation of antibody diversity. Cell 1990;60:963–970.

54   Reynaud CA, Garcia C, Hein WR, Weill JC: Hypermutation generating the sheep immunoglobulin repertoire is an antigen independent process. Cell 1995;80:115–125.

55   Lebecque SG, Gearhart PJ: Boundaries of somatic mutation in rearranged immunoglobulin genes: 5″ boundary is near the promoter, and 3′ boundary is ~1 Kb from V-D-J gene. J Exp Med 1990; 172:1717–1727.

56   Yelamos J, Klix N, Goyenechea B, Lozano F, Chui WL, Gonzalez-Fernandez A, Pannell R, Neuberger MS, Milstein C: Targeting of non-Ig sequences in place of the V segment by somatic hypermutation. Nature 1995;376:225–229.

57   Peters A, Storb U: Somatic hypermutation of Ig genes is linked to transcription initiation. Immunity 1996;4:57–65.

58   Lee S, Elenbaas B, Levine A, Griffith J: P53 and its 14 Kd C terminal domain recognize primary DNA damage in the form of insertion/deletion mismatches. Cell 1995;81:1013–1020.

Dr. V. Pascual, Department of Microbiology, University of Texas Southwestern Medical Center, Dallas, TX 75235-9140 (USA)

Ferrarini M, Caligaris-Cappio F (eds): Human B Cell Populations.
Chem Immunol. Basel, Karger, 1997, vol 67, pp 58–69

....

Subepithelial B Cells of the Human Tonsil

Mariella Dono[a], *Simona Zupo*[a], *Carlo E. Grossi*[b, c], *Nicholas Chiorazzi*[d], *Manlio Ferrarini*[a, e]

[a] Servizio di Immunologia Clinica, Istituto Nazionale per la Ricerca sul Cancro (IST),
[b] Istituto di Anatomia Umana dell'Università di Genova,
[c] Servizio di Patologia Clinica, IST, Genova, Italy;
[d] Departments of Medicine, North Shore University Hospital and New York
University School of Medicine, Manhasset, N.Y., USA;
[e] Department of Experimental and Clinical Oncology, Università di Genova, Genova,
Italy

In secondary lymphoid organs, B cells are organized predominantly in defined structures, i.e. secondary follicles which consist of a germinal center (GC) surrounded by a follicular mantle (FM) [1, 2]. B cells that proliferate in the GC undergo a concomitant process of hypermutation of VH and VL genes [3, 4]. Subsequently, the cells that express Ig receptors of high affinity for the stimulating antigen are facilitated in their clonal expansion, whereas B cells with Ig receptors of irrelevant or even self-specificity or of low affinity for the stimulating antigen are eliminated [3, 5, 6]. Deletion of the unwanted B cells occurs by apoptosis [6].

FM B cells are comprised primarily of virgin B cells which express surface IgM and IgD and other surface markers [detected by monoclonal antibodies (mAb)] different from those of GC B cells [7–10]. Although the relationships between the two types of follicular B cells are far from clear, recent evidence has indicated that, upon antigenic stimulation, certain FM B cells can reach the GC and transform into GC B cells.

Another subset of B cells, distinct from both FM and GC B cells, is comprised of the so-called extrafollicular B cells [11]. The prototypic example of this subset is represented by the B cells of the splenic marginal zone (MZ) [12–14], although, in man, B cells of the tonsillar subepithelial (SE) area, of the inner surface of the marginal sinus of lymph nodes, of the thymic medulla and of the dome region of the Peyer's patches are considered to belong to the same B cell subpopulation [15–18]. The splenic MZ, defined as the outermost area of the white pulp that surrounds secondary follicles, is populated by IgM+ IgD–, nonrecirculating B cells [19]. These cells are characterized by the ability of responding to T-independent type 2 (TI-2) antigens [20, 21]. Traditionally, TI antigens are subdivided into two groups: TI-1 antigens that are lipopolysaccharides and TI-2 antigens that are polysaccharides with repeated epitopes. TI-2 antigens are poorly degradable in vivo and elicit long-lasting responses of the IgM isotype [21].

In a series of experiments aimed at characterizing different B cell subsets from human tonsils, we were able to isolate homogeneous suspensions of B cells that were phenotypically and functionally distinct from both GC and FM B cells. Subsequent observations revealed that this 'novel' B cell subset was comprised of SE B cells. According to a topographical definition, tonsillar SE B cells are located in the lamina propria, underneath the epithelium that lines the tonsil surface above and between the lymphoid follicles. Lymphocytes that infiltrate the tonsil squamous epithelium, particularly in the depth of the cryptae, also appear to belong to this subset. The availability of purified tonsillar SE B cells allowed us to carry out a number of functional studies which, indeed, demonstrated their striking similarity with splenic MZ B cells [22, 23].

In this review, we shall summarize these data and also anticipate some preliminary studies on the structure of their VH genes which indicate that SE B cells may be comprised of both nonmutated and mutated B cells.

Isolation of a Subset of B Cells Identified as SE B Cells

The initial observation that led to the purification of SE B cells was that the high density B cells collected at the interface between 100 and 60% discontinuous Percoll gradients were heterogeneous and could be further fractionated into two distinct subsets according to the expression of surface CD5 (see fig. 1). While CD5+ B cells had the typical surface phenotype of FM B cells (see fig. 1), CD5– B cells had a surface phenotype not only distinct from that of FM B cells, but also from that of GC B cells collected in Percoll fractions of lower density (fig. 1). The phenotype of CD5– B cells shown in figure 1 is similar to that reported for extrafollicular B cells in a number of different human tissues. These similarities are reinforced by the observation that, like other extrafollicular B cells [11], CD5– B cells have low to absent expression of CD21, CD23, CD24, CD75 and CD77. Moreover, unlike FM B cells that express both IgM and IgD [11], CD5– B cells have high density surface IgM and low density surface IgD, and are virtually negative for IgG and IgA. Finally, cells with the same phenotype as tonsillar CD5– B cells are not detected in the peripheral blood, another result that is in accord with the contention that extrafollicular B cells do not recirculate, but are part of a resident B cell pool [19].

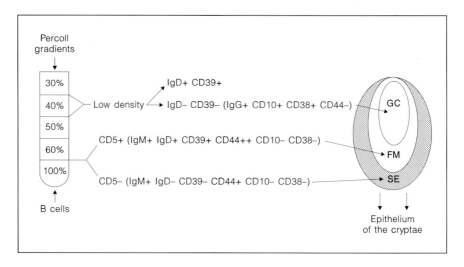

Fig. 1. A correlate between purified B cell subsets and their anatomical localization. Purified B cells from tonsils were fractionated on Percoll density gradients. The high density cells layered between 100 and 60% Percoll fractions were collected and further separated into two subsets on the basis of CD5 expression. The low density cells obtained by pooling the cells present in the 30 and 40% Percoll fractions were depleted of cells expressing IgD and CD39. The three resulting populations were stained with a panel of mAb in indirect immunofluorescence and analyzed by flow cytometry. In situ immunohistochemical studies performed on tonsil sections revealed that the B cells with identical phenotype of the B cell subsets obtained in suspensions could be detected in three different anatomical areas: FM zone, SE area, and GC of the follicle.

Comparison of the surface phenotype of CD5– B cells in suspension with that of the SE B cells determined in situ revealed an almost complete identity. The region beneath the epithelial cryptae was largely populated by B cells and by a few macrophages, T cells and plasma cells. The majority of the B cells expressed low to absent levels of CD10, CD21, CD22, CD23, CD24, CD38 and CD77. Unlike that observed in cell suspensions, the in situ staining demonstrated that some SE B cells expressed CD39. These apparent discrepancies, however, could have been the result of the different state of activation of the two cell populations analyzed. Thus, while CD5– B cells isolated in suspension were resting cells as assessed by cell cycle flow-cytometric analysis and by spontaneous ^{3}H thymidine incorporation, the SE B cells were also comprised of activated cells as documented by the expression of CD69 in certain cells. In this connection, it is perhaps worth recalling that CD39 expression by B cells may be a function of the state of cell activation. The concept that tonsillar SE areas are populated by both resting and activated B cells is also in agreement with the observation that, in this site, plasma cells are relatively numerous, possibly indicating an active stimulation by antigens penetrating through the tonsillar epithelial linings.

Ultrastructural and Histochemical Studies

The ultrastructural analysis of SE B cells in situ and of CD5– B cells in suspensions demonstrated that the two cell types had identical morphology. These B cells displayed an extended endosomal compartment and a characteristic organization of the chromatin that was distributed in small packets which conferred a speckled appearance to the nucleus (fig. 2). This nuclear morphology was not observed in GC or FM B cells. In addition, FM B cells had a much higher nuclear/cytoplasmic ratio, while GC B cells were blast-like cells (centroblasts) or large cells with indented nuclei (centrocytes). Notably, ultrastructural in situ studies revealed that SE areas also contained activated lymphocytes, macrophages and plasma cells, thus confirming the aforementioned concept that this is an area of active cell stimulation.

Studies on the cytochemical localization of alkaline phosphatase activity provided data for further similarities between SE B cells in situ and CD5– B cells in suspensions. In fact, alkaline phosphatase activity was detected in a large proportion of the SE B cells analyzed in situ or in suspension, whereas it was virtually absent in both GC and FM B cells.

Functional Differences between SE B Cells and FM or GC B Cells

The capacity of producing polyreactive antibodies has been traditionally considered a distinguishing feature of FM B cells [23], while the ability of undergoing spontaneous apoptosis in vitro is a characteristic property of GC B cells [24]. The absence of these two functions from SE B cells could therefore be taken as evidence for further differences between SE and GC or FM cells. Indeed, studies in which highly purified SE or FM B cells were infected with EBV and subsequently expanded in vitro showed that only the cell lines derived from FM B cells were capable of producing antibodies to rheumatoid factor, anti-ds or ss-DNA reactivity (taken as the prototypic examples of polyreactive antibodies). In contrast, in a variety of different experimental conditions the capacity to undergo spontaneous apoptosis in vitro was detected only in suspensions of highly purified GC B cells, and not in SE B cells.

The observation that SE B cells displayed an extended endosomal compartment together with their localization in areas readily exposed to antigens pene-

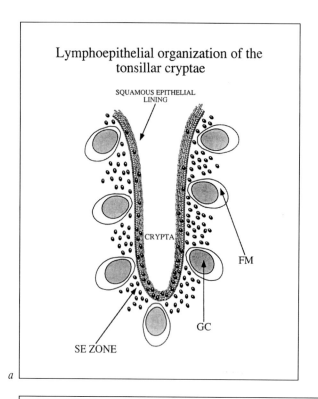

Lymphoepithelial organization of the
tonsillar cryptae

SQUAMOUS EPITHELIAL
LINING

CRYPTA

FM

GC

SE ZONE

a

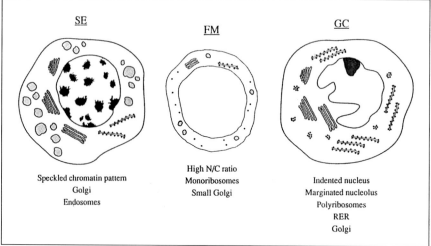

SE

FM

GC

Speckled chromatin pattern
Golgi
Endosomes

High N/C ratio
Monoribosomes
Small Golgi

Indented nucleus
Marginated nucleolus
Polyribosomes
RER
Golgi

b

Fig. 2. a A schematic representation of a tonsillar crypta surrounded by secondary lymphoid follicles with large GC. Lymphocytes are abundant in the lamina propria and also populate the squamous epithelium. *b* Major ultrastructural features of lymphoid cells that are predominant in the SE zone, in FM and in GC. RER = Rough endoplasmic reticulum.

trating through the epithelial lining of the tonsils suggested that perhaps SE B cells could be endowed with good antigen-presenting capacities. Due to obvious experimental difficulties posed by the use of tonsillar cells, this hypothesis could not be tested directly in assays of specific antigen presentation.

However, it is generally assumed that the stimulatory ability of a cell in mixed leukocyte reactions (MLR) provides an estimate of its antigen-presenting capacities. Therefore, irradiated SE B cells were cocultured with neonatal or adult T cells and the proliferation of the latter cells was subsequently measured by ^{3}H thymidine incorporation. SE B cells were capable of inducing a good proliferative response of both neonatal (potentially capable of mounting primary responses only) and adult (capable of primary as well as secondary responses) T cells. The stimulatory capacity of SE B cells was almost as efficient as that of dendritic cells purified from the peripheral blood. Notably, however, SE B cells had to be activated with anti-μ-ab in order to become good MLR stimulators. This was not surprising since SE B cells purified in suspension did not express the costimulatory molecules CD80 and CD86; exposure of SE B cells to anti-μ-ab induced the expression of CD80 and CD86. These antigens were clearly involved in the activation of the MLR as documented by the finding that the presence in culture of anti-CD80 and CD86 mAb resulted in a substantial inhibition of the MLR. In connection with this, it is of interest that Liu et al. [25] have recently described a subset of tonsillar B cells that share several characteristics with the SE B cells described here, including their topographical location underneath or within the tonsillar epithelium. These cells, called memory B cells for their predominant expression of surface IgG, elicited MLR without need for preactivation by anti-μ-ab, a finding that was also consistent with their constitutive expression of CD80 and CD86. These cells also expressed other activation markers such as CD95 not found on the SE B cells studied by us. It is conceivable that the two populations of cells described here and by Liu et al. [25] represent two different stages of activation of the same B cell subset. Indeed, preliminary data on tonsillar B cells from low density Percoll gradient fractions have demonstrated the presence of cells with features of activated SE B cells.

FM B cells were also tested in parallel for their capacity to elicit an MLR by both neonatal and adult T cells. A proliferative response was noticed with both types of responders when FM B cells were preactivated with anti-μ-ab, although its magnitude was consistently lower than that observed with SE B cells. Thus, these observations establish another substantial difference between the functional features of SE and FM B cells.

Analysis of Ig VH4 Genes Indicates that SE B Cells Are Comprised of Both Virgin and Memory B Cells

Previous functional studies conducted primarily in rats indicated that the splenic MZ B cells are comprised of both memory and virgin B cells [26]. The functional approach employed in the experimental animal models could not be obviously used for human cells. However, implications about this issue could be derived from the sequence analysis of the VH region genes used by these cells. As alluded to earlier, B cells undergo point mutations of their VH and VL region genes in the GC and there is a subsequent selection of those cells that have developed antibodies of higher affinity for the stimulating antigen.

Analyses of the IgH variable region genes were carried out by sequencing 18 rearranged IgM transcripts from isolated SE B cells of two separate tonsils. To estimate the rate of somatic mutations, the sequences obtained were compared with the corresponding germline sequences. The gene segment usage among the VH4 segments was random with a slight increase of VH4-34 (VH4.21) usage in the second tonsil sample analyzed. Clonally related transcripts were rarely found. The rate of somatic mutation indicated that approximately a half of the sequenced clones were mutated with similarity to the corresponding germline genes ranging from 94 to 100%. In half of the studied clones, analyses of replacement to silent mutation ratios within the CDRs and the FRs supported an active role for antigen selection. In the other half, these replacement mutations were uniformly distributed between the CDR and the FR. Altogether these data suggest that the SE B cells are comprised of three different populations: one without significant VH mutations, one with significant replacement mutations that are localized predominantly in the CDRs, and one with replacement mutations spread throughout the VH gene (fig. 3). These may indicate the presence of nonmutated, perhaps virgin B cells that have not yet encountered antigen or B cells that have encountered antigen in a T cell-independent fashion that does not promote V gene mutation.

Whether selection of memory SE B cells occurs in the GC or perhaps directly within the SE areas is still an unresolved problem. In this connection it is of interest that the memory cells described by Pascual et al. [7], that were alluded to before, also display accumulations of point mutations in the V region genes utilized by their IgM and IgG molecules. These findings raise questions regarding their relationship with the SE B cells described here. One possibility is that those cells that bear IgM molecules represent activated progenitors of our IgM+ SE B cells, as suggested by their expression of activation markers. If this were the case, one could speculate that, in the absence of a continuous antigenic stimulation, those activated B cells revert to resident, quiescent SE B cells. Notably, in this regard, we find very few if any IgG+ SE B cells and have considerable difficulties

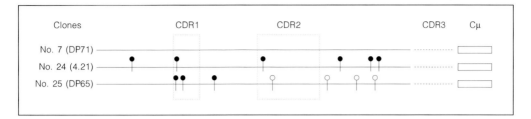

Fig. 3. VH4 sequences from SE B cells. Each line represents one molecular clone. On the left the clone number and the corresponding germline sequence are indicated. Mutations are represented by replacement mutation (● with stem) and silent mutation (○ with stem). CDR1 and CDR2 sequences are boxed. The sequence analysis indicated three different patterns of mutations in the VH4 genes of SE B cells: clone No. 7 is unmutated, clone No. 24 shows replacement mutations throughout the VH gene and clone No. 25 has significant mutations in the CDR region. The three different clones were derived from the same tonsil specimen.

in isolating IgG mRNA from our resting CD5– B cell fractions. Collectively, these data perhaps suggest a partial or complete incapacity of cells that have switched over to isotypes other than IgM to become quiescent, memory SE B cells. It remains to be seen whether this is related to the fact that these activated IgG+ B cells differentiate into the numerous plasma cells found in the SE area, or whether they migrate to different lymphoid areas.

Response of SE B Cells to Antigens and Mitogens

A variety of experimental and clinical observations have demonstrated that the splenic MZ is the site where the responses to TI-2 antigens take place [20, 21, 27, 28]. Due to their similarities with the splenic MZ B cells, we also tested whether tonsillar SE B cells were able to respond to TI-2 antigens. For these experiments, we used TNP-Ficoll as a typical TI-2 antigen, while TNP-*Brucella abortus* was employed as TI-1 antigen. The antibody-producing cells formed in culture in response to either antigens were measured by a sensitive ELI spot assay. Collectively, these experiments indicated that (1) SE B cells could respond to TI-2 but not to TI-1 antigens, (2) this response occurred only if IL2 (but not other lymphokines such as IL3, IL5, IL6, IL10) was present, a finding which is in line with previous results showing that TI-2 responses require the indirect assistance of T cells, and (3) this response occurred in the absence of macrophages or of other accessory cells. The latter finding would support the notion that the capacity to respond to TI-2 antigens is an intrinsic property of SE B cells and shed some light on the long-lasting controversy of whether the MZ B cells or their microenvironment is primarily responsible for the good TI-2 responses observed in this particular area.

These experiments also showed that the ability to mount TI-2 responses is a unique feature of SE B cells, since no other cell subset among those obtained by fractionation of tonsillar B cells on Percoll gradients was capable of mounting this response. Notably, also the B cells from the peripheral blood failed to respond to TI-2 antigens, thus reinforcing the aforementioned concept that SE B cells are nonrecirculating B cells.

The capacity of SE B cells to respond to TI-2 antigens in the complete absence of accessory cells was in striking contrast with their inability to respond to a variety of polyclonal B cell activators. These included SAC and anti-μ-ab in the presence or absence of cytokines, and also CD40L or CD40 mAb with IL2 or IL4 and/or anti-μ-ab in various combinations [8, 9]. Although somehow unexpected, these findings support further the contention that tonsillar SE B cells belong to the extrafollicular B cell subpopulation. Recent experiments aimed at isolating murine MZ B cells have determined that they are characterized by a good response to TI-2 antigens together with a poor to absent response to a variety of polyclonal B cell activators. Like the SE B cells described here, murine MZ B cells express high levels of surface IgM and low to absent surface IgD and CD23. It is of interest that SE B cells, although incapable of proliferating or producing IgM antibodies or even of undergoing apoptosis, nevertheless become activated in response to polyclonal B cell activators as documented by their enlarged size and by the expression of a variety of surface activation markers. Collectively, these data suggest that SE B cells need to be signalled through particular surface structures in order to progress into the cell cycle or to differentiate into Ig-secreting plasma cells. This notion would also be in line with the observation that the close contact with activated T cells drives SE B cells into both proliferation and Ig secretion. This experimental system appears to be particularly suitable for attempts to define the surface structures necessary for SE B cells to interact with T cells and to be subsequently activated. This is particularly true considering that not only human but also murine T cells can activate SE B cells. This latter observation opens up several possibilities for experimental approaches in which murine mAb to human B cell surface structures are employed to inhibit T-B interactions. Studies along this line are currently in progress.

Concluding Remarks

Our studies demonstrate that the human tonsils represent a suitable source of SE B cells that can be purified in suspension and also used for functional studies. The data so far collected have indicated that these cells share functional, phenotypic and trafficking characteristics consistent with those of extrafollicular B cells obtained from other sources, both in man and in other animal species. Considering the current difficulties in obtaining specimens of human lymphoid tissues, the tonsils may well become the major source of material for studies on extrafollicular B cells.

Although SE B cells appear phenotypically and functionally different from both of the other cell subsets (FM and GC) also isolated from tonsillar tissue, there are not yet clear indications as to their relationships. Our findings show that SE B cells are comprised of both virgin and memory B cells. This appears even more true if one also considers the observations of Liu et al. [25], who have described a subset of subepithelial B cells that have switched over to IgG and have the features of memory B cells as determined by VH and VL region sequencing. Since accumulation of point mutations and selection together with isotype switches occur primarily in the GC, it is plausible that upon stimulation by antigen (presumably entering into tonsils through its epithelial lining), virgin SE B cells become activated and move to GC where they complete their process of differentiation into memory B cells before moving again to the subepithelial area. According to this hypothesis, SE B cells would thus pass through a stage of GC or GC-like cells.

Likewise, the relationship between FM and SE B cells is far from clear. Traditionally, FM B cells have been considered as being comprised of virgin B cells endowed with the capacity to actively recirculate. In man, support for this hypothesis is provided both by the V gene sequence work and by the observation that peripheral blood B cells have the phenotype of FM B cells. Since SE B cells, like all extrafollicular B cells, are resident cells, these considerations would suggest that the two cell subsets belong to completely distinct populations. However, additional options should be considered. For example, the newly formed B cells exiting from the bone marrow are a single cell subset which will be driven into differentiation into one of the mature subpopulations depending upon the environment where the cell happens to home. Or else, there are several distinct subpopulations of young B cells destined to accomplish different maturation programs. If the second hypothesis holds true, then we have to consider the existence of B cells with an FM-like phenotype that are committed to become SE B cells. Likewise, it is known that extrafollicular B cells can leave their homing site to enter the circulating cell pool from where they can reexit to home into another appropriate site (i.e. from the tonsillar SE area to the mucosa-associated lymphoid tissue). During this period in the circulation, do the SE B cells maintain their original phenotype and perhaps choose some specific routes that include the lymphatic circulation? Or else, do these cells acquire, perhaps temporarily, the phenotypic features of FM B cells? These and several other problems related to B cell subset populations are now amenable to experimental analysis owing to the possibility of purifying the various B cell subsets.

References

1 Liu YJ, Johnson GD, Gordon J, MacLennan ICM: Germinal centres in T-cell-dependent antibody responses. Immunol Today 1992;13:17–21.
2 Thorbecke GJ, Amin AR, Tsiagbe VK: Biology of germinal centers in lymphoid tissue. FASEB J 1994;8:832–840.
3 Berek C, Berger A, Apel M: Maturation of the immune response in germinal centers. Cell 1991;67: 1121–1129.
4 Jacob J, Kelsoe G, Rajewsky K, Weiss U: Intraclonal generation of antibody mutants in germinal centres. Nature 1991;354:389–392.
5 Nossal GJV: The molecular and cellular basis of affinity maturation in the antibody response. Cell 1992;68:1–5.
6 Liu YJ, Joshua DE, Williams GT, Smith CA, Gordon J, MacLennan ICM: Mechanism of antigen-driven selection in germinal centres. Nature 1989;324:929–931.
7 Pascual V, Liu YJ, Magalski A, De Bouteiller O, Banchereau J, Capra D: Analysis of somatic mutation in five B cell subsets of human tonsil. J Exp Med 1994;180:329–339.
8 Dono M, Zupo S, Masante R, Taborelli G, Chiorazzi N, Ferrarini M: Identification of two distinct CD5– B cell subsets from human tonsils with different responses to CD40 monoclonal antibody. Eur J Immunol 1993;23:873–881.
9 Zupo S, Dono M, Azzoni L, Chiorazzi N, Ferrarini M: Evidence for differential responsiveness of human CD5+ and CD5– B cell subsets to T cell-independent mitogens. Eur J Immunol 1991;21: 351–359.
10 Kuppers R, Zhao M, Hansmann ML, Rajewsky K: Tracing B cell development in human germinal centres by molecular analysis of single cells picked from histological sections. EMBO J 1993;12: 4955–4967.
11 Möller P, Mielke B: Extrafollicular peripheral B-cell report; in Knapp W, et al (eds): Leukocyte Typing. IV. White Cell Differentiation Antigens. Oxford, Oxford University Press, 1989, pp 213–215.
12 Times W, Poppema S: Lymphocyte compartments in human spleen. An immunohistologic study in normal spleens and uninvolved spleens in Hodgkin's disease. Am J Pathol 1985;120:443–454.
13 Gray D, McConnell I, Kumararatne DS, MacLennan IC, Humphrey JH, Bazin H: Marginal zone B cells express CR1 and CR2 receptors. Eur J Immunol 1984;14:47–52.
14 Dunn Walters DK, Isaacson PG, Spencer J: Analysis of mutations in immunoglobulin heavy chain variable region genes of microdissected marginal zone (MGZ) B cells suggests that the MGZ of human spleens is a reservoir of memory B cells. J Exp Med 1995;182:559–566.
15 Morente M, Piris MA, Orradre JL, Rivas C, Villuendas R: Human tonsil intraepithelial B cells: Marginal zone-related subpopulation. J Clin Pathol 1992;45:668–672.
16 van der Oord JJ, de Wolf-Peeters C, Desmet VJ: The marginal zone in the human reactive lymph node. Am J Clin Pathol 1986;86:475–479.
17 Möller P, Mielke B, Hofmann WJ: Immunophenotype of medullary thymic B-cells; in Knapp W, et al (eds): Leukocyte Typing. IV. White Cell Differentiation Antigens. Oxford, Oxford University Press, 1989, pp 222–224.
18 Spencer J, Finn T, Pulford KAF, Mason DY, Isaacson PG: The human gut contains a novel population of B lymphocytes which resemble marginal zone cells. Clin Exp Immunol 1985;62:607–612.
19 Gray D, MacLennan IC, Bazin H, Khan M: Migrant mu+ delta+ and mu+ delta– B lymphocyte subsets. Eur J Immunol 1982;12:564–572.
20 Amlot PI, Grennan D, Humphrey JH: Splenic dependence of the antibody response to thymus-independent (TI-2) antigens. Eur J Immunol 1985;15:508–512.
21 Mosier DE, Subbarao B: Thymus independent antigens: Complexity at B-lymphocyte activation revealed. Immunol Today 1982;3:217.
22 Dono M, Burgio VL, Tacchetti C, Favre A, Augliera A, Zupo S, Taborelli G, Chiorazzi N, Grossi CE, Ferrarini M: Subepithelial B cells in the human palatine tonsil. I. Morphologic, cytochemical and phenotypic characterization. Eur J Immunol 1996;26:2035–2042.

23 Dono M, Zupo S, Augliera A, Burgio VL, Massara R, Melagrana A, Costa M, Grossi CE, Chiorazzi N, Ferrarini M: Subepithelial B cells in the human palatine tonsil. II. Functional characterization. Eur J Immunol 1996;26:2043–2049.
24 Zupo S, Rugari E, Dono M, Taborelli G, Malavasi F, Ferrarini M: CD38 signaling by agonistic monoclonal antibody prevents apoptosis of human germinal center B cells. Eur J Immunol 1994;24: 1218–1222.
25 Liu Y-J, Barthelemy C, de Bouteiller O, Arpin C, Durand I, Banchereau J: Memory B cells from human tonsils colonize mucosal epithelium and directly present antigen to T cells by rapid upregulation of B7.1 and B7.2. Immunity 1995;2:239–254.
26 MacLennan ICM, Chan E: The dynamic relationship between B-cell populations in adults. Immunol Today 1993;14:29–33.
27 Timens W, Boes A, Rozeboom Uiterwijk T, Poppema S: Immaturity of the human splenic marginal zone in infancy. Possible contribution to the deficient infant immune response. J Immunol 1989; 143:3200–3206.
28 Amlot PL, Heyes AE: Impaired human antibody response to the thymus-independent antigen, DNP-Ficoll, after splenectomy. Implications for post-splenectomy infections. Lancet 1985;iv: 1008–1011.

Dr. Mariella Dono, Istituto Nazionale per la Ricerca sul Cancro, IST,
Servizio di Immunologia Clinica, Largo Rosanna Benzi, n. 10, 16132 Genova GE (Italy)

Ferrarini M, Caligaris-Cappio F (eds): Human B Cell Populations.
Chem Immunol. Basel, Karger, 1997, vol 67, pp 70–84

....

Malignant Lymphomas Stem from Different B Cell Populations

Philip M. Kluin, J. Han, J.M. van Krieken

Department of Pathology, Leiden University Hospital, Leiden, The Netherlands

Lymphoproliferative disorders comprise approximately 30 different sub-types which include leukemias of precursor B or T cells, chronic leukemias of (im)mature B or T cells, non-Hodgkin's lymphomas (NHL), (multiple) myeloma/ plasmacytoma and Hodgkin's disease. Recently, all entities have been redefined and listed by an international group of pathologists, resulting in the Revised European American Lymphoma (REAL) classification [1]. Since the introduction of monoclonal antibody technology, cytogenetics and molecular genetics, classification of lymphoproliferative disorders is increasingly based on biological aspects of tumor cells.

From a theoretical point of view, lymphoproliferative disorders can be classi-fied in two different ways: (1) classification based on the genetic origin of the tumor cells, taking into account the genetic abnormalities in tumor (precursor) cells, and (2) classification according to the morphology and phenotype of accu-mulating tumor cells. The latter is the classical way of classification as developed in the 1970s, and it follows the concept of the 'frozen stage model'. For B cell neoplasias, a variation on this theme is characterization of tumor cells according to the pattern of rearrangements and especially mutations within immunoglobu-lin genes at 14q32. In normal lymphoid tissues, both Ig class switching and hyper-mutations within the IgH genes at 14q32 are concentrated within the follicle cen-ters. Extensive studies of the Rajewsky group [2] in Cologne with help of single cell PCR and sequencing have demonstrated that normal mantle zone cells are devoid of hypermutations, whereas normal follicle center cells continuously undergo extensive hypermutations within these Ig genes. These hypermutations may result in amino acid replacements. Replacements at the antigen binding sites of the molecules, the complementary determining regions (CDRs) may influence binding affinity to antigen. The occurrence of random hypermutations and selection of subclones with the highest affinity to the antigen is an important mechanism in affinity maturation. Therefore, the presence of ongoing hypermutations in Ig genes (as evidenced by sequence analysis of Ig genes obtained from multiple B cells or subclones) may be used as a marker of follicle center cells. Postfollicle center cells will be marked by mutations as well, but they do not undergo ongoing mutations. Additionally, overrepresentation of certain amino acid sequences within the CDRs by conservation of similar replacement mutations or of germline sequences as compared to framework regions may be used as a marker of antigenic selection.

At present many molecular biologists, pathologists and clinicians tend to claim that genetic classification as shown in figure 1, is more solid than morphologic and phenotypic classification. In contrast to phenotypic analysis, genetic analysis may disclose the 'roots' of a certain tumor. Indeed in many malignancies with a relatively simple genetic constellation, a genetic abnormality (like a translocation) may hint at an early and essential genetic event in tumorigenesis without which the tumor could not develop. An example is the t(11;14) in mantle cell lymphoma by which cyclin D1 is overexpressed. Such an abnormality can be used as a 'genetic marker' for diagnosis. In mantle cell lymphoma the recognition of this translocation and in consequence overexpression of cyclin D1 protein have greatly improved our accuracy of diagnosis. The relevance of genetic markers is best illustrated in acute myeloid leukemia in which genetic classification is nowadays more relevant than classification according to the morphologic French-American-British classification system.

On the other hand, the phenotypic approach has the great theoretical advantage that the phenotype is the cumulative result of all genetic and other hits that affected the tumor cells and their precursor cells. Most if not all tumors arise after accumulation of multiple (genetic) alterations, and these genetic alterations may differ in their contribution to the biology of tumor cells. Statistically, the biological relevance of individual genetic abnormalities may decline with an increase in the overall complexity of genetic abnormalities. In many carcinomas it is often very difficult if not impossible to trace the earliest genetic events that affected tumor precursor cells and to trace the genetic events that are most relevant to the behavior of the tumor. Moreover, events that are essential in early cancerogenesis may have lost their significance later on. For instance, (1) early loss of DNA repair function may allow other genetic events to lead to a fully malignant tumor, and (2) the role of the Epstein-Barr virus in the pathogenesis of the African-type Burkitt's lymphoma may be taken over by chromosomal translocation t(8;14) and activation of MYC. Therefore, it is understandable that simple clinical parameters like lymph node status in breast cancer (in fact a surrogate marker for accu-

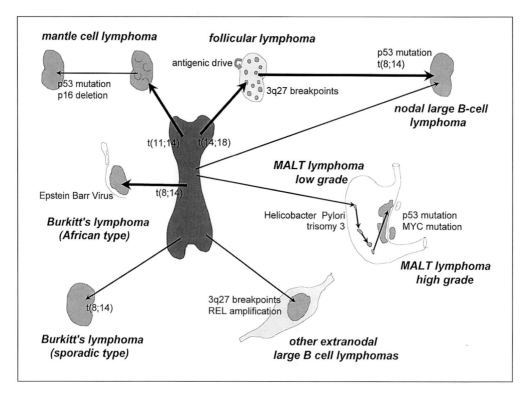

Fig. 1. Origin of B cell lymphoma. A simplified scheme of the genetic origin of the currently identified, major genetic events in B cell lymphoma is shown. In mantle cell lymphoma, follicular lymphoma and African Burkitt's lymphoma, characteristic translocations occur in bone marrow-derived precursor B cells (thick arrows, bone marrow shown as a bone). In these lymphomas, the site of origin of these translocations and the actual site of presentation of clinical disease are different. So far, no such early translocations have been identified in other lymphomas (thin arrows). In these lymphomas, translocations and other mutations may occur later on, and possibly at the site of clinical presentation. In follicular lymphoma, mantle cell lymphoma and MALT lymphoma, additional events like p53 mutation may cause tumor progression. This is associated with a 'large cell' morphology.

mulated genetic damage) are of more prognostic relevance than individual genetic abnormalities in multivariate analyses. As will be discussed later on, large B cell lymphomas may represent lymphomas with a similar complex genetic makeup.

Another drawback of the genetic approach is that some lymphoproliferative entities lack a recurrent chromosomal abnormality that gives a clue to their origin. An example is hairy cell leukemia: a combination of morphology with the immunophenotype of tumor cells (CD19 or other pan-B cell marker, CD11c, CD25 plus

CD103) is unique for this type of malignancy, but we do not know anything of the tumorigenesis and genetic events in this particular neoplasm.

Finally, it should be noted that a translocation characteristic for a distinct type of lymphoma occasionally may be found in an 'unrelated' tumor type with a different phenotype. The classical example of such a promiscuous abnormality is the t(9;22). Production of classical p190 chimeric BCR-ABL protein as found in chronic myeloid leukemia is also identified in approximately half of the acute lymphocytic leukemias with t(9;22). Most likely, the occurrence of additional genetic events early after the occurrence of t(9;22) results into this phenotypic divergence.

In this chapter we will review the current knowledge of the genesis of certain B cell lymphomas, mantle cell lymphoma, follicular lymphoma, Burkitt's lymphoma and large B cell lymphoma.

Mantle Cell Lymphoma

Mantle cell lymphoma is a recently redefined entity [1, 3], and represents approximately 5% of all NHL. Previously, mantle cell lymphoma was called centrocytic lymphoma in the Kiel classification [4], and described as intermediately differentiated lymphocytic lymphoma, intermediate lymphocytic lymphoma or mantle zone lymphoma in the American literature [5, 6]. Patients with this disease have a poor outcome with a median survival of 2–3 years [7]. Mantle cell lymphoma shows a monotonous accumulation of small to intermediately sized lymphoid cells with more or less cleaved nuclei, easily leading to confusion with centrocytes of the follicle center lymphomas or lymphocytes in chronic lymphocytic leukemia (CLL). Mantle cell lymphoma has a characteristic phenotype: the tumor cells invariably show strong surface IgM staining, often with coexpression of IgD, lack cytoplasmic Ig expression, and are almost always CD5+, CD10– and CD23–. This phenotype distinguishes mantle cell lymphoma from follicle center cell lymphomas that are CD5– and CD10+, from lymphocytic lymphomas/CLL that are CD23+, and from marginal zone lymphomas that are CD5– and CD10– [8]. However, although characteristic, the phenotype of mantle cell lymphoma is not unique and not present in 100% of cases.

Like normal IgM+ IgD+ mantle zone and circulating blood B cells, mantle cell lymphoma and CLL lack hypermutations [in rare IgG expressing CLLs mutations have been described, 9]. This indicates that the accumulating cells have not entered the follicle center cell reaction (prefollicle center B cells). Also like CLL, mantle cell lymphoma expresses CD5. In men, there is no evidence that CD5-positive B cells represent a distinct lineage, and hence, there is also no indication that mantle cell lymphoma and CLL are derived from a distinct B cell subset.

Most if not all mantle cell lymphomas carry a t(11;14)(q13;q32) with a breakpoint within the B cell lymphoma 1 (BCL-1) region at 11q13. Applying interphase fluorescence in situ hybridization and especially the novel DNA fiber fluorescence in situ hybridization assay to released DNA molecules enabling simultaneous detection and mapping of breakpoints in large genomic regions, we demonstrated 11q13 breakpoints in approximately 95% of all mantle cell lymphomas. These breakpoints are scattered over a region of at least 220 kb [10]. Molecular analysis of the 11q13 and 14q32 breakpoints strongly suggests that the translocations occur early as an error during D-J or V-DJ recombination in bone marrow precursor B cells [11, 12]. In a minority of patients variant translocations like t(2;11)(p11;q13) or t(11;22)(q13;q12) involve Ig light chain loci [13]. The target gene at 11q13 is cyclin D1/CCND1, previously called PRAD1. Due to the t(11;14) and juxtaposition to the Eμ enhancer, cyclin D1 will be constitutively expressed in IgH-expressing B cells. Type D1, D2 and D3 cyclins play an essential role in the regulation of the cell cycle, especially in the transition from the G1 into the S phase. In normal lymphoid cells, cyclin D2 and D3 but not cyclin D1 are used. Type D cyclins seems to be redundant since all types can complex with CDK4. What is the effect of t(11;14) and overexpression of cyclin D1 in B cells? One explanation may be that normal mantle zone cells have a relatively low expression of cyclin D2 and D3 expression; in consequence, overexpression of cyclin D1 in this specific phase of B cell maturation may give these cells a certain growth advantage over normal B cells.

Rare variant-type CLLs with an increase of prolymphocytes, splenic lymphomas with villous lymphocytes [14–16], and rare myelomas [17, 18] also carry a t(11;14) and may overexpress cyclin D1. Cyclin D1 overexpression without apparent translocation is also regularly observed in hairy cell leukemia [19, 20]. The molecular mechanisms and additional genetic events involved in these cases have not been elucidated. The 'promiscuous' presence of t(11;14) and cyclin D1 expression in B cell neoplasias other than mantle cell lymphoma underlines the danger to use a single genetic event as a tumor marker.

In mantle cell lymphoma, additional events like p53 mutations and p16 deletions may supervene t(11;14). Some studies indicate that these additional abnormalities are associated with a blastic or pleomorphic cellular morphology and with extremely poor survival [21–24].

Follicular Lymphoma

Follicular lymphoma represents 20% of all NHL in Europe. It is characterized by the accumulation of follicle center B cells, centroblasts and centrocytes. Both, the degree of follicularity and the relative number of centroblasts (the proliferating cells) can vary between and within individual tumors. Phenotypically, follicular lymphoma cells are mature B cells with the expression of surface IgM, IgG or IgA. Interestingly, some IgM tumors coexpress IgD, a feature not seen in normal follicle center B cells. Like normal follicle B cells, almost all follicular lymphomas express CD10 and are CD5 negative. Also like normal follicles, the presence of numerous reactive CD4+ T cells and of follicular dendritic cells suggests that the tumor cells depend on environmental factors, perhaps antigen, for survival and proliferation.

The hypothesis that growth of follicular lymphoma cells depends on antigen is also supported by the very high frequency of ongoing hypermutations and the dominance of certain amino acid replacement mutations within the CDRs [25, 26]. The lack of IgH expression in approximately 5% of these lymphomas can be explained by hypermutations resulting in stop codons. This suggests that some follicular lymphomas may have become antigen-independent.

The clonal advantage of follicular lymphoma cells over normal B cells is explained by the constitutive expression of the BCL-2 protein caused by the translocation t(14;18)(q32;q21). As shown by Korsmeyer [27], the BCL-2 protein is a member of a large family of proteins involved in positive and negative regulation of apoptosis. Constitutive expression of BCL-2 in B and T cells of transgenic mice and transfected cell lines results in enhanced cell survival and resistance to many signals that normally induce programmed cell death like irradiation and exposure to cytotoxic drugs [28–30]. Like t(11;14), the t(14;18) has its origin in an aberrant D-J or V-DJ recombination in early precursor B cells [31–33]. The selective effect of this translocation and BCL-2 expression on cell survival much later on during maturation in follicle center B cells is explained by the fact that normal follicle center B cells downregulate BCL-2. This leads to extensive cell death of normal centrocytes. Neoplastic centrocytes with t(14;18) continue to express BCL-2 and hence selectively survive during this phase of B cell maturation.

Based on the selective survival of t(14;18) carrying B cells and the observation that follicular lymphoma cells have antigen-driven patterns of IgH mutations, one might consider a two-hit model for follicular lymphoma: a combination of t(14;18) leading to enhanced cell survival and antigen recognition leading to proliferation may be sufficient for lymphoma genesis. Two observations strongly oppose this simple model: (1) transgenic mice with constitutive expression of BCL-2 in all B cells do not develop follicular lymphoma but only mild lymphoid hyperplasia [34], and (2) as demonstrated by our and other groups, many normal individuals (more than 50%) carry large numbers (1 in 10^5 or more) of t(14;18) positive B cells but do not develop lymphoma [35–37]. These observations suggest that more (genetic?) events are necessary to drive these t(14;18) cells to follicular lymphoma.

Most follicular lymphomas show a distinct block in maturation: the tumor cells do not or occasionally differentiate into plasma cells [38]. Apparently, signals to drive the cells further to plasma cells are absent. However, such a differentiation may occasionally be observed. We described a patient with follicular lymphoma who showed a dramatic but transient maturation into plasma cells caused by treatment with IL3 and simultaneous induction of very high levels of endogenous IL6 [39]. This transient life of the blockage also dramatically changed the clinical picture of the patient: the patient developed transient myeloma/plasma cell leukemia with paraproteinemia and Bence Jones proteinuria. In the literature, occasional cases of multiple myeloma with a t(14;18) and especially t(11;14) with deregulation of cyclin D1 have been described [17, 18, 40]. Theoretically, these cases might represent B cell neoplasia in which the normally present maturation blocks have been overthrown by maturation-inducing factors.

Additional genetic events may follow t(14;18). One event is the t(8;14)(q24;32) also occurring in Burkitt's lymphoma [41]. This translocation can occur immediately after the t(14;18) giving rise to a precursor blasts crisis with the expression of terminal transferase [42]. More commonly, the event gives rise to a mature phenotype (Burkitt's or large B cell type; see below). Other events are mutations in p53, and alterations in 3q27 affecting the BCL-6 gene (see below). As demonstrated by several groups, p53 mutations may play an important role in the progression to large B cell lymphoma [43, 44]. The role of BCL-6 rearrangements in these tumors is puzzling [45]. Apparently, they do not result in any increase of aggressiveness.

Although the t(14;18) is characteristic of follicular lymphoma or progressed follicular lymphoma, variant translocations involving BCL-2 at 18q21 may occur in an unrelated malignancy, i.e. B-CLL. In 5–10% of CD5-positive B-CLL, a breakpoint 5′ of BCL-2 may occur [46–48]. As demonstrated by Adachi et al. [46, 47], Ig light chain genes at chromosome 2 or 22 instead of the heavy chain gene complex at chromosome 14q32 may function as a chromosomal partner.

Burkitt's Lymphoma

In Western countries, Burkitt's lymphoma represents approximately 5% or less of all NHL. It is characterized by an extremely high proliferation rate of relatively small blast cells. Morphologically and immunophenotypically, Burkitt's lymphoma cells look like small centroblasts. Therefore, it has been claimed that Burkitt's lymphoma cells represent the malignant counterpart of early blasts normally detectable in the early phase of the follicle center cell reaction.

From an epidemiologic point of view, at least two different types of Burkitt's lymphoma can be distinguished: the African type and non-African type. Both may represent ends of a spectrum. African or endemic Burkitt's lymphoma arises in a context of malaria infection, undernourishment and Epstein-Barr infection. Similar cases may occur in some HIV-infected patients in the western world. Non-African, nonendemic or sporadic cases arise in patients without these risk factors in western countries. The prototype is a large ileocecal mass in children. The vast majority of AIDS-related Burkitt's, lymphomas in western countries are also EBV-negative and are of this type. Another type that morphologically mimics Burkitt's lymphoma is the so-called 'non-Burkitt's, small noncleaved lymphoma'. This type may represent secondary progressed lymphomas with a Burkitt's-like morphology; the relatively older age and the high frequency of t(14;18) normally associated with follicular lymphoma [49, 50] support this view.

One study on hypermutations in Ig genes in 6 African-type Burkitt's lymphoma cell lines showed extensive hypermutations indicating that the cells indeed represent follicle center or postfollicle center cells. In one of these cell lines mutation patterns in the CDRs indicated real antigen selection [50, 51].

Most if not all Burkitt's lymphomas carry translocations affecting MYC at 8q24. The most common translocation is t(8;14)(q24;32). Variant types involve the IgL genes at chromosomes 2 and 22. Similar to mantle cell lymphoma and follicular lymphoma, African types of breakpoints may involve the JH or DH genes at 14q32 or the IgL genes at 2p21 and 22q11, indicating an early origin in precursor B cells. In contrast, in sporadic Burkitt's lymphoma breakpoints are more common at Sμ and Sα at 14q32, indicating an origin of mature class switching B cells. Within the 8q24 region, breakpoints may be found within or immediately 5′ of MYC, far 5′ and far (several hundreds of kb) 3′ of MYC. Some but no strict association between JH and DH recombinations at 14q32 with distant 5′ MYC recombinations in African Burkitt's lymphoma versus Sμ and Sα recombinations at 14q32 with nearby 5′ or intronic MYC recombinations at 8q24 in sporadic cases have been identified [52, 53]. The latter type is reminiscent of the translocations that can be found in pristane-induced plasmacytomas in mice [54]. Other variant translocations associated with a different geographic origin of Burkitt's lymphoma have been described [55].

As for cyclin D1 and BCL-2, experiments in transfected cell lines and transgenic mice, but also in pristane-induced plasmacytomas in mice indicate that deregulation of MYC itself is insufficient for transformation. This is supported by observations that B cells with a MYC-Sμ or MYC-Sα recombination indicating a t(8;14) can be identified in normal and HIV-infected individuals by PCR [56].

Large B Cell Lymphoma

Large B cell lymphomas represent 30–40% of all NHL. Large B cell lymphomas are characterized by a diffuse growth of large B cell blasts. Cytomorphologically, 4 different types of centroblasts, pleomorphic or anaplastic centrocytes, immunoblasts and plasmablasts, may be present. Approximately half of the large B cell lymphomas arise within lymph nodes, the other half at extranodal sites like the stomach, small and large bowel, skin, thyroid, testis, soft tissues, or brain. Interestingly, most extranodal sites lack any preexistent lymphoid tissue. One hypothesis to explain the genesis of these lymphomas is that they are preceded by chronic inflammation leading to induction of lymphoid tissue. Such a scenario is currently accepted for lymphoma of the stomach [57]. *Helicobacter pylori* infecton may induce chronic inflammation, which in turn may induce the formation of mucosa-associated lymphoid tissue (MALT). A low-grade lymphoma derived from the so-called parafollicular B cells may develop within this induced MALT and subsequently may progress to high-grade MALT lymphoma, a subtype of large B cell lymphoma (fig. 1). In other large B cell lymphomas no such origin from preexistent lymphoid tissue or preexistent low-grade lymphoma can be documented.

Large B cell lymphomas are very heterogeneous in clinical aspects, especially dissemination patterns. For instance nodal lymphomas tend to spread to other lymph nodes, tonsil, and bone marrow, MALT lymphoma to locoregional lymph nodes or other MALT sites, testicular lymphoma to the contralateral testis and cerebrum, and bone lymphoma to other skeletal sites. Most likely these patterns reflect the presence of specific adhesion molecules involved in invasion, circulation, or adherence to endothelial cells [58, 59].

Different genetic abnormalities have been reported in large B cell lymphomas, but they have not been systematically analyzed in relationship to clinical presentation, especially site of presentation. They consist of chromosomal translocations, numerical abnormalities, amplifications, deletions and point mutations. Only recently, attention was paid to the possible involvement of tumor suppressor genes in the genesis of these lymphomas.

So far the most frequent breakpoint in large B cell lymphoma is at the BCL-6 gene at 3q27. Breakpoints are found in approximately 25–35% of cases, including AIDS-related large B cell lymphomas [60–63]. In contrast to breakpoints within BCL-1, BCL-2 and MYC, BCL-6 breakpoints seem to be clustered in a small region of 10 kb. BCL-6 breakpoints are not unique for large B cell lymphomas and also occur in 10–15% of follicular lymphomas where they may coexist with t(14;18) [45]. No breakpoints were found in mantle cell lymphoma or Burkitt's lymphoma. The BCL-6 gene, also called LAZ-3 [64] and BCL-5 [65] by other groups, codes for a novel zinc-finger protein, with homology to Drosophila transcription factors. By translocation it is juxtaposed to a large number of different translocation partners. In consequence BCL-6 has been called a 'promiscuous gene'. Only in less than 50% of cases is the IgH locus a partner. Within the IgH locus the breakpoint usually is at a switch recombination site and not at JH or DH, suggesting that these recombinations are relatively late and secondary events. The biological and clinical significance of BCL-6 rearrangements in large B cell lymphoma is unknown. One group claimed an association with extranodal disease and a relatively very good prognosis [66]. However, this could not be confirmed by other groups [61].

The second most frequent translocation in large B cell lymphoma is the t(14;18) with a breakpoint within BCL-2. This translocation is present in approximately 15% of cases. Interestingly, it is almost absent from primary extranodal large B cell lymphoma, and completely absent from extranodal large B cell lymphoma arising within the MALT [67, 68]. Most likely, t(14;18)-positive large B cell lymphomas represent progressed follicular lymphomas. Like the occurrence of a blast crisis in CML, progression may occur late during disease and after presentation of follicular lymphoma, but it may also occur earlier during the subclinical phase of the disease; in the latter case, the patient will present with a de novo t(14;18) large B cell lymphoma. Also interestingly and unlike the situation in follicular lymphoma, there is almost no correlation between the presence of t(14;18) and expression of BCL-2 protein in large B cell lymphoma: approximately 50% of large B cell lymphomas express BCL-2 protein, but only 15% harbor a translocation; furthermore, approximately one third of large B cell lymphomas with a t(14;18) do not express the protein.

The third most common translocation in large B cell lymphoma is the t(8;14) with involvement of MYC at 8q24. As determined by banding analysis and Southern blot analysis, the frequency is approximately 5–10% [66, 67, 69]. Possibly, most breakpoints are 5′ or in the first intron of MYC, and at IgH switch sites of 14q32. In some large B cell lymphomas a combination of t(14;18) and t(8;14) has been identified, and the molecular analysis of these cases suggests that the t(8;14) is secondary to the t(14;18) [41].

Translocations t(11;14) involving the 11q13 region have only be rarely detected in large B cell lymphomas. Four large B cell lymphomas with a t(11;14) and additional deletion of p16 have been reported recently by Koduru et al. [21]. As already discussed, mantle cell lymphomas with secondary p53 mutation often have a so-called anaplastic or pleomorphic morphology; this subtype of mantle cell lymphoma is difficult to distinguish from large B cell lymphoma using morphology alone [22–24]. On the other hand, we tested large B cell lymphomas for cyclin D1 overexpression and identified only 2 positive cases in a large series of more than 200 large B cell lymphomas. This suggests that progression of t(11;14)-carrying mantle cell lymphoma to large B cell lymphoma is extremely rare.

Other chromosomal and molecular genetic abnormalities, including complex abnormalities, are frequently found in large B cell lymphoma. In a recent report a high frequency of amplification at 2p including the REL gene was found for primary extranodal large B cell lymphoma [70, 71], especially mediastinal large B cell lymphoma [72]. These (primary thymic?) B cell lymphomas have a unique clinical behavior with bulky local tumor growth, and late extranodal dissemination.

A remarkable observation may shed additional light on the genesis of large B cell lymphomas. Patterns of Ig gene hypermutations have not been regularly studied in large B cell lymphomas, however, in one study a skewed VH gene usage was found with a predominance of VH4 in 15/17 large B cell lymphomas, in particular the VH4.21 gene [73]. The use of this gene is associated with cold agglutinin disease and binding specificity for the i/I carbohydrate antigen on erythrocytes. In contrast, a normal distribution of VH genes was found in follicular lymphoma. If this finding is confirmed in larger series, it might suggest that some large cell lymphomas have a common origin, or that lymphomas with a particular VH gene usage (and antigen recognition?) have a propensity to transform to large cell lymphomas.

Conclusions

Over the past 10 years combined immunophenotypical analysis and molecular studies on the configuration of the Ig genes and chromosomal translocations have brought new insight into the genesis and evolution of many B cell lymphomas. The absence or presence of ongoing or stable hypermutations in IgH genes indicates a blocking of B cell maturation at distinct stages of B cell maturation, respectively, before, during or after the follicle center cell formation. Specific patterns of replacement mutations in CDRs, as well as selective VH gene usage hint at antigen-driven proliferation or antigen specificity.

In follicular lymphoma, mantle cell lymphoma and African Burkitt's lymphoma, a multistep pathogenesis includes the occurrence of a chromosomal translocation arising very early within bone marrow precursor B cells, followed by unidentified other (genetic) events. Follicular and mantle cell lymphoma may subsequently progress by developing additional genetic abnormalities like p53 mutation. In other lymphomas, for instance lymphocytic lymphoma, immunocytoma and MALT lymphomas, characteristic translocations are absent or so far unidentified.

The clinically heterogeneous large B cell lymphomas contain variable and often complex genetic abnormalities, and form a genetic wastebasket. This wastebasket can only be sorted out by multiparameter analysis of large series of lymphomas, especially taking into account the primary site of presentation and dissemination of the lymphoma.

References

1　Harris NL, Jaffe ES, Stein H, Banks PM, Chan JKC, Cleary ML, Delsol G, De Wolf-Peeters C, Falini B, Gatter KC, Grogan TM, Isaacson PG, Knowles DM, Mason DY, Muller-Hermelink H-K, Pileri SA, Piris MA, Ralfkiaer E, Warnke RA: A revised European-American classification of lymphoid neoplasms: A proposal from the International Lymphoma Study Group. Blood 1994;84: 1361–1392.

2　Jacob J, Kelsoe G, Rajewsky K, Weiss U: Intraclonal generation of antibody mutants in germinal centres. Nature 1991;354:389–392.

3　Banks PM, Chan J, Cleary ML, Delsol G, De Wolf-Peeters C, Gatter K, Grogan TM, Harris NL, Isaacson PG, Jaffe ES, Mason D, Pileri S, Ralfkiaer E, Stein H, Warnke RA: Mantle cell lymphoma: A proposal for unification of morphologic, immunologic, and molecular data. Am J Surg Pathol 1992;16:637–640.

4　Lennert K, Feller AC: Histopathologie der Non-Hodgkin-Lymphome. Springer Semin Immunopathol 1990; pp 91–99.

5　Duggan MJ, Weisenburger DD, Ye YL, Bast MA, Pierson JL, Linder J, Armitage JO: Mantle zone lymphoma: A clinicopathologic study of 22 cases. Cancer 1990;66:522–529.

6　Weisenburger DD, Duggan MJ, Perry DA, Sanger WG, Armitage JO: Non-Hodgkin's lymphomas of mantle zone origin. Pathol Ann 1991;26:139–158.

7　Velders GA, Kluin-Nelemans JC, De Boer CJ, Hermans J, Noordijk EM, Schuuring E, Kramer MHH, van Deijk WA, Rahder JB, Kluin PM, Van Krieken JHJM: Mantle cell lymphoma: A population based clinical study. J Clin Oncol 1996;14:1269–1274.

8　Zucca E, Stein H, Coiffier B: European Lymphoma Task Force (ELTF): Report of the Workshop on Mantle Cell Lymphoma (MCL). Ann Oncol 1994;5:507–511.

9　Ebeling SB, Schutte MEM, Logtenberg T: Molecular analysis of V_H and V_L regions expressed in IgG-bearing chronic lymphocytic leukemia (CLL): Further evidence that CLL is a heterogeneous group of tumors. Blood 1993;82:1626–1631.

10　Vaandrager JW, Schuuring E, Zwikstra E, De Boer CJ, Kleiverda JK, Van Krieken JHJM, Kluin-Nelemans JC, Van Ommen GJB, Raap AK, Kluin PM: Direct visualization of dispersed 11q13 chromosomal translocations in mantle cell lymphoma by multi-color DNA fiber FISH. Blood 1996; 88:1177–1182.

11　Tsujimoto Y, Yunis JJ, Onorato-Showe L, Erikson J, Nowell PC, Croce CM: Molecular cloning of the chromosomal breakpoint of B-cell lymphomas and leukemias with the t(11;14) chromosome translocation. Science 1984;224:1403–1406.

12　Tsujimoto Y, Louie E, Bashir MM, Croce CM: The reciprocal partners of both the t(14;18) and the t(11;14) translocations involved in B-cell neoplasms are rearranged by the same mechanism. Oncogene 1988;2:347–351.

13　Komatsu H, Lida S, Yamamoto K, Mikuni C, Nitta M, Takahashi T, Ueda R, Seto M: A variant chromosome translocation at 11q13 identifying PRAD1/cyclin D1 as the BCL-1 gene. Blood 1994; 84:1226–1231.

14　Cuneo A, Balboni M, Piva N, Rigolin GM, Roberti MG, Mejak C, Moretti S, Bigoni R, Balsamo R, Cavazzini P, et al: Atypical chronic lymphocytic leukaemia with t(11;14)(q13;32): Karyotype evolution and prolymphocytic transformation. Br J Haematol 1995;90:409–416.

15　Delmer A, Ajchenbaum-Cymbalista F, Tang R, Ramond S, Faussat AM, Marie JP, Zittoun R: Over-expression of cyclin D1 in chronic B-cell malignancies with abnormality of chromosome 11q13. Br J Haematol 1995;89:798–804.

16　Jadayel D, Matutes E, Dyer MJS, Brito-Babapulle V, Khokhar MT, Oscier D, Catovsky D: Splenic lymphoma with villous lymphocytes: Analysis of BCL-1 rearrangements and expression of the cyclin D1 gene. Blood 1994;83:3664–3671.

17　VandenBerghe H, Vermaelen K, Louwagie A, Criel A, Mecucci C, Vaerman J-P: High incidence of chromosome abnormalities in IgG3 myeloma. Cancer Genet Cytogenet 1984;11:381–387.

18　Fiedler W, Weh HJ, Hossfeld DK: Comparison of chromosome analysis and BCL-1 rearrangement in a series of patients with multiple myeloma. Br J Haematol 1992;81:58–61.

19　De Boer CJ, Kluin-Nelemans JC, Dreef EJ, Kester MGD, Kluin PM, Schuuring E, Van Krieken JHJM: Involvement of the CCND1 gene in hairy cell leukemia. Ann Oncol 1996;7:251–256.

20 Bosch F, Campo E, Jares P, Pittaluga S, Munoz J, Nayach I, Piris MA, De Wolf-Peeters C, Jaffe ES, Rozman C, Montserrat E, Cardesa A: Increased expression of the PRAD-1/CCND1 gene in hairy cell leukemia. Br J Haematol 1995;91:1025–1030.

21 Koduru PRK, Zariwala M, Soni M, Gong JZ, Xiong Y, Broome JD: Deletion of cyclin dependent kinase 4 inhibitor genes p15 and p16 in non-Hodgkin's lymphoma. Blood 1995;86:2900–2905.

22 Louie DC, Offit K, Jaslow R, Parsa NZ, Murty VV, Schluger A, Chaganti RS: p53 overexpression as a marker of poor prognosis in mantle cell lymphomas with t(11;14)(q13;q32). Blood 1995;86:2892–2899.

23 Hernandez L, Fest T, Cazorla M, Teruya-Feldstein J, Bosch F, Peinado MA, Piris MA, Montserrat E, Cardesa A, Jaffe ES, Campo E, Raffeld M: p53 gene mutations and protein overexpression are associated with aggressive variants of mantle cell lymphoma. Blood 1996;87:3351–3359.

24 Greiner TC, Moynihan MJ, Chan WC, Lytle DM, Pedersen A, Anderson JR, Weisenburger DD: p53 mutations in mantle cell lymphoma are associated with variant cytology and predict a poor prognosis. Blood 1996;87:4302–4310.

25 Zelenetz AD, Chen TT, Levy R: Clonal expansion in follicular lymphoma occurs subsequent to antigenic selection. J Exp Med 1992;176:1137–1148.

26 Bahler DW, Levy R: Clonal evolution of a follicular lymphoma: Evidence for antigen selection. Proc Natl Acad Sci USA 1992;89:6770–6774.

27 Korsmeyer SJ: Bcl-2 initiates a new category of oncogenes: Regulators of cell death. Blood 1992;80:879–886.

28 Walton MI, Whysong D, O'Connor PM, Hockenbery D, Korsmeyer SJ, Kohn KW: Constitutive expression of human Bcl-2 modulates nitrogen mustard and camptothecin induced apoptosis. Cancer Res 1993;53:1853–1861.

29 Hockenbery DM, Oltvai ZN, Yin XM, Milliman CL, Korsmeyer SJ: BCL-2 functions in an antioxidant pathway to prevent apoptosis. Cell 1993;75:241–251.

30 Miyashita T, Reed JC: Bcl-2 oncoprotein blocks chemotherapy-induced apoptosis in a human leukemia cell line. Blood 1993;81:151–157.

31 Bakhshi A, Jensen JP, Goldman P, Wright JJ, McBride OW, Epstein AL, Korsmeyer SJ: Cloning the chromosomal breakpoint of t(14;18) human lymphomas: Clustering around Jh on chromosome 14 and near a transcriptional unit on 18. Cell 1985;41:899–906.

32 Tsujimoto Y, Gorham J, Cossman J, Jaffe E, Croce CM: The t(14;18) chromosome translocations involved in B-cell neoplasms result from mistakes in VDJ joining. Science 1985;229:1390–1393.

33 Cleary ML, Sklar J: Nucleotide sequence of a t(14;18) chromosomal breakpoint in follicular lymphoma and demonstration of a breakpoint-cluster region near a transcriptionally active locus on chromosome 18. Proc Natl Acad Sci USA 1985;82:7439–7443.

34 McDonnell TJ, Deane N, Platt FM, Nunez G, Jaeger U, McKearn JP, Korsmeyer SJ: bcl-2-immunoglobulin transgenic mice demonstrate extended B cell survival and follicular lymphoproliferation. Cell 1989;57:79–88.

35 Limpens J, Stad R, Vos C, de Vlaam C, De Jong D, Van Ommen GJB, Schuuring E, Kluin PM: Lymphoma associated translocation t(14;18) in blood B cells of normal individuals. Blood 1995;85:2528–2536.

36 Limpens J, De Jong D, Van Krieken JHJM, Price CGA, Young BD, Van Ommen G-JB, Kluin PM: Bcl-2/JH rearrangements in benign lymphoid tissues with follicular hyperplasia. Oncogene 1991;6:2271–2276.

37 Liu Y, Hernandez AM, Shibata D, Cortopassi GA: BCL2 translocation frequency rises with age in humans. Proc Natl Acad Sci USA 1994;91:8910–8914.

38 Keith TA, Cousar JB, Glick AD, Vogler LB, Collins RD: Plasmacytic differentiation in follicular center cell (FCC) lymphomas. Am J Clin Pathol 1985;84:283–290.

39 Kramer MH, Kluin PM, Wijburg ER, Fibbe WE, Kluin-Nelemans HC: Differentiation of follicular lymphoma cells after autologous bone marrow transplantation and haematopoietic growth factor treatment. Lancet 1995;345:488–490.

40 Nishida K, Taniwaki M, Misawa S, Abe T: Nonrandom rearrangement of chromosome 14 at band q32.33 in human lymphoid malignancies with mature B-cell phenotype. Cancer Res 1989;49:1275–1281.

41   Yano T, Jaffe ES, Longo DL, Raffeld M: MYC rearrangements in histologically progressed follicular lymphomas. Blood 1992;80:758–767.
42   De Jong D, Voetdijk BMH, Beverstock GC, Ommen van GJB, Willemze R, Kluin PhM: Activation of the c-*myc* oncogene in a precursor-B-cell blast crisis of follicular lymphoma, presenting as composite lymphoma. N Engl J Med 1988;318:1373–1378.
43   Lo Coco F, Gaidano G, Louie DC, Offit K, Chaganti RSK, Dalla-Favera R: P53 mutations are associated with histologic transformation of follicular lymphoma. Blood 1993;82:2289–2295.
44   Sander CA, Yano T, Clark HM, Harris C, Longo DL, Jaffe ES, Raffeld M: P53 mutation is associated with progression in follicular lymphoma. Blood 1993;82:1994–2004.
45   Otsuki T, Yano T, Clark HM, Bastard C, Kerckaert JP, Jaffe ES, Raffeld M: Analysis of LAZ3 (BCL-6) status in B-cell non-Hodgkin's lymphomas: Results of rearrangement and gene expression studies and a mutational analysis of coding region sequences. Blood 1995;85:2877–2884.
46   Adachi M, Cossman J, Longo D, Croce CM, Tsujimoto Y: Variant translocation of the bcl-2 gene to immunoglobulin lambda light chain gene in chronic lymphocytic leukemia. Proc Natl Acad Sci USA 1989;86:2771–2774.
47   Adachi M, Tefferi A, Greipp PR, Kipps TJ, Tsujimoto Y: Preferential linkage of BCL-2 to immunoglobulin light chain gene in chronic lymphocytic leukemia. J Exp Med 1990;171:559–564.
48   Raghoebier S, Van Krieken JHJM, Kluin-Nelemans JC, Gillis A, Van Ommen GJB, Ginsberg AM, Raffeld M, Kluin PhM: Oncogene rearrangements in chronic B-cell leukemia. Blood 1991;77:1560–1564.
49   Yano T, Van Krieken JHJM, Magrath IT, Longo DL, Jaffe ES, Raffeld M: Histogenetic correlations between subcategories of small noncleaved cell lymphomas. Blood 1992;79:1282–1290.
50   Tamaru J, Hummel M, Marafioti T, Kalvelage B, Leoncini L, Minacci C, Tosi P, Wright D, Stein H: Burkitt's lymphomas express VH genes with a moderate number of antigen-selected somatic mutations. Am J Pathol 1995;147:1398–1407.
51   Chapman CJ, Mockridge CI, Rowe M, Rickinson AB, Stevenson FK: Analysis of VH genes used by neoplastic B cells in endemic Burkitt's lymphoma shows somatic hypermutation and intraclonal heterogeneity. Blood 1995;85:2176–2181.
52   Neri A, Barriga F, Knowles DM, Magrath IT, Dalla-Favera R: Different regions of the immunoglobulin heavy-chain locus are involved in chromosomal translocations in distinct pathogenetic forms of Burkitt lymphomas. Proc Natl Acad Sci USA 1988;85:2748–2752.
53   Magrath I: The pathogenesis of Burkitt's lymphoma. Adv Cancer Res 1990;55:133–270.
54   Janz S, Müller J, Shaughnessy J, Potter M: Detection of recombinations between c-myc and immunoglobulin switch α in murine plasma cell tumors and preneoplastic lesions by polymerase chain reaction. Proc Natl Acad Sci USA 1993;90:7351–7365.
55   Shiramizu B, Barriga F, Neequaye J, Jafri A, Dalla-Favera R, Neri A, Guttierez M, Levine P, Magrath I: Patterns of chromosomal breakpoint locations in Burkitt's lymphoma: Relevance to geography and Epstein-Barr virus association. Blood 1991;77:1516–1526.
56   Müller JR, Janz S, Goedert JJ, Potter M, Rabkin CS: Persistence of immunoglobulin heavy chain/C-MYC recombination-positive lymphocyte clones in the blood of human immunodeficiency virus-infected homosexual men. Proc Natl Acad Sci USA 1995;92:6577–6581.
57   Isaacson PG: Is gastric lymphoma an infectious disease? Hum Pathol 1993;24:569–570.
58   Horst E, Meijer CJLM, Radaszkiewicz T, Ossekoppele GJ, Van Krieken JHJM, Pals ST: Adhesion molecules in the prognosis of diffuse large-cell lymphoma: Expression of a lymphocyte homing receptor (CD44), LFA-1 (CD11a/18), and ICAM-1 (CD54). Leukemia 1990;4:595–599.
59   Joensuu H, Ristamäki R, Klemi PJ, Jalkanen S: Lymphocyte homing receptor (CD44) expression is associated with poor prognosis in gastrointestinal lymphoma. Br J Cancer 1993;68:428–432.
60   Ye BH, Lista F, Lo Coco F, Knowles DM, Offit K, Chaganti RSK, Dalla-Favera R: Alterations of a zinc finger-encoding gene, BCL-6, in diffuse large-cell lymphoma. Science 1993;262:747–750.
61   Bastard C, Deweindt C, Kerckaert JP, Lenormand B, Rossi A, Pezzella F, Fruchart C, Duval C, Monconduit M, Tilly H: LAZ3 rearrangements in non-Hodgkin's lymphoma: Correlation with histology, immunophenotype, karyotype, and clinical outcome in 217 patients. Blood 1994;83:2423–2427.

62   Pescarmona E, Lo Coco F, Pacchiarotti A, Rapanotti MC, Cimino G, Di Paolo B, Baroni CD: Analysis of the BCL-6 gene configuration in diffuse B-cell non-Hodgkin's lymphomas and Hodgkin's disease. J Pathol 1995;177:21–25.

63   Gaidano G, Lo Coco F, Ye BH, Shibata D, Levine AM, Knowles DM, Dalla-Favera R: Rearrangements of the BCL-6 gene in acquired immunodeficiency syndrome-associated non-Hodgkin's lymphoma: Association with diffuse large-cell subtype. Blood 1994;84:397–402.

64   Kerckaert J-P, Deweindt C, Tilly H, Quief S, Lecocq G, Bastard C: LAZ3, a novel zinc-finger encoding gene, is disrupted by recurring chromosome 3q27 translocations in human lymphomas. Nature Genet 1993;5:66–70.

65   Miki T, Kawamata N, Hirosawa S, Aoki N: Gene involved in the 3q27 translocation associated with B cell lymphoma, BCL5, encodes a Krüppel-like zinc-finger protein. Blood 1994;83:26–32.

66   Offit K, Lo Coco F, Louie DC, Parsa NZ, Leung D, Portlock C, Ye BH, Lista F, Filippa DA, Rosenbaum A, et al: Rearrangement of the bcl-6 gene as a prognostic marker in diffuse large-cell lymphoma. N Engl J Med 1994;331:74–80.

67   Raghoebier S, Kramer MHH, Van Krieken JHJM, De Jong D, Limpens J, Kluin-Nelemans JC, Van Ommen GJB, Kluin PM: Essential differences in oncogene involvement between primary nodal and extranodal large cell lymphoma. Blood 1991;78:2680–2685.

68   Jacobson JO, Wilkes BM, Kwiatkowski DJ, Medeiros LJ, Aisenberg AC, Harris NL: bcl-2 rearrangements in de novo diffuse large cell lymphoma: Association with distinctive clinical features. Cancer 1993;72:231–236.

69   Ladanyi M, Offit K, Jhanwar SC, Filippa DA, Chaganti RSK: MYC rearrangement and translocations involving band 8q24 in diffuse large cell lymphomas. Blood 1991;77:1057–1063.

70   Lu D, Thompson JD, Gorski GK, Rice NR, Mayer MG, Yunis JJ: Alterations at the rel locus in human lymphoma. Oncogene 1991;6:1235–1241.

71   Houldsworth J, Mathew S, Rao PH, Dyomina K, Louie DC, Parsa N, Offit K, Chaganti RS: REL proto-oncogene is frequently amplified in extranodal diffuse large cell lymphoma. Blood 1996;87: 25–29.

72   Joos S, Otaño-Joos MI, Ziegler S, Brüderlein S, Du Manoir S, Bentz M, Möller P, Lichter P: Primary mediastinal (thymic) B-cell lymphoma is characterized by gains of chromosomal material including 9p and amplification of the REL gene. Blood 1996;87:1571–1578.

73   Hsu FJ, Levy R: Preferential use of the VH4 Ig gene family by diffuse large cell lymphoma. Blood 1995;86:3072–3082.

Philip M. Kluin, Department of Pathology, Leiden University Hospital, PO Box 9600,
NL–2300 RC Leiden (The Netherlands)
Tel. 31-71-5266592/5266624, Fax 31-71-5248158,
E-mail: p.m.kluin@pathology.medfac.leidenuniv.nl

Ferrarini M, Caligaris-Cappio F (eds): Human B Cell Populations.
Chem Immunol. Basel, Karger, 1997, vol 67, pp 85–101

....

What Do Chronic B Cell Malignancies Teach Us about B Cell Subsets?

O. Pritsch[a], *K. Maloum*[b], *C. Magnac*[a], *F. Davi*[b], *J.L. Binet*[b],
H. Merle-Béral[b], *G. Dighiero*[a]

[a] Unité d'Immuno-hématologie et d'Immunopathologie, Institut Pasteur et
[b] Département d'Hématologie, CHU Pitié-Salpêtrière, Paris, France

During recent years, considerable progress has been made in understanding B cell physiology. Phenotypic, functional and immunoglobulin (Ig) gene expression studies contributed new and relevant information to the understanding of B cell biology. In this work, we review the available evidence concerning the existence of different B cell subsets and the contribution of human B cell malignancies to the better understanding of this question.

B Cell Lineages

In mice, Ly1-B cell (CD5+ B cells) [1, 2] have been postulated to correspond to distinct B cell subsets. The CD5 marker, initially reported to identify a T helper subset [3], was subsequently shown to be a pan-T cell marker and to be also present on a small subpopulation of murine B cells [4]. This subpopulation accounts for 1–2 and 5–10% of splenocytes in BALB/c and NZB mouse, respectively. They are largely predominant among the peritoneal B cell population (20–40% in BALB/c and 40–80% in NZB) [5].

Phenotypically, CD5+ B cells are characterized by high surface IgM expression and low expression of membrane IgD and B220 (CD45), expressed along with most well-known B cell markers [1, 2]. During ontogeny, CD5+ B cells predominate in the fetus and neonate [1, 6, 7]. Work, mainly carried out in Herzenberg's lab [1], indicated that CD5+ B cells can survive longer in culture than CD5– B cells but they cannot be reconstituted in lethally irradiated mice with adult bone marrow cells. In contrast, CD5– B cells express IgM dull, IgD and CD45 bright, are reconstituted by bone marrow-derived B cells and do not ensure self-replenishment. These experiments suggest a different origin for CD5+ B cells [8, 9]. This point has been supported by evidence, showing a paucity of nontemplated N region sequence insertions at the VHDH and DHJH junctions [10, 11]. Such rearrangements are typical of those made by early fetal B cells, before the developmental expression of terminal deoxynucleotidyltransferase (TdT), responsible for N insertions in the junctions. These results suggest that adult CD5+ B cells may have undergone Ig gene rearrangement and differentiation during early B cell ontogeny. Furthermore Ly1-B cells may be involved mainly in the production of autoantibodies [12].

Several findings are in agreement with the latter assumption: (1) there is increased frequency of CD5-positive B cells in NZB [5] and moth-eaten autoimmune prone strains [13], (2) a lack of CD5+ B cells parallels a lack of autoantibody secretion in CBA/N Xid mice [2, 5], (3) increased frequency of CD5+ B cells in newborn mice is in agreement with the increased frequency of natural autoantibodies (NAAB) precursors, as observed by somatic hybridization [14, 15], (4) an increased frequency of CD5+ B cells in the peritoneal cavity [5] parallels an increased frequency of antibromelinated mouse red blood cell activity in this particular compartment [16] and (5) there is a restricted V gene expression among CD5+ B cells from peritoneal cavity [10–17].

However, some discrepancies concerning CD5+ B cells and autoantibody production exist. (1) The lupus-prone mouse strain MRL lpr/lpr does not exhibit a high frequency of CD5+ B cells [18, 19]. (2) Xid mice, known because they do not express the CD5 marker on B cells, display a frequency of NAAB precursors similar to that observed in non-Xid mice [20]. (3) The frequency of NAAB precursors in the peritoneal cavity enriched in CD5+ B cells has not been found to be any higher than that observed with the splenic repertoire in which CD5+ B cells constitute a minor population, excepted for antibromelinated mouse red blood cell activity [21]. (4) A study based on the detection of the mRNA transcript of the CD5 gene by Northern blotting among hybridomas with NAAB specificity derived from several mouse strains indicated that NAAB arise from both CD5+ and CD5– B lymphocyte subsets [22].

Although this hypothesis was attractive, recent work in both human and murine models challenged the idea that CD5+ B cells could constitute a separate lineage since (1) CD5+ B cells proliferating in chronic lymphocytic leukemia (CLL) are expressing low amounts of membrane IgM [23], (2) results from reconstitution experiments could not be consistently reproduced, (3) CD5– B cells can be induced to gain CD5 following treatment with anti-μ and IL-6, which suggests the possibility that CD5 could constitute an activation marker [24, 25], (4) CD5– B cells are also producing autoantibodies [20, 26] and (5) restricted usage of V genes has only been substantiated in the case of mouse peritoneal cavity CD5+ B cells [10, 17].

In an expert meeting [27, 28], a new nomenclature for CD5+ and CD5– B cells was proposed. Because the CD5 marker may not be detected in B cells sharing properties with CD5+ B cells and this marker may be induced [24] in CD5– B cells, it was argued that CD5 may not be the right marker to define these subpopulations. Thus, CD5+ cells were segregated into B1a cells, initially defined by the expression of CD5 marker characterized by IgM^{hi}, IgD^{lo}, CD45^{lo}, Mac1+, IL-5R+ and FcεR– which differs from that displayed by conventional B cells (B-2; IgM^{lo}, IgD^{hi}, CD45^{hi}, Mac1–, IL-5R– and FcεR+) [27]. A third B cell subset, B1b cells, also identified in mice displays a pattern of cell surface markers and functional properties similar to the B1a population but does not express the CD5 marker [27, 28]. Each of these subsets has been proposed to represent different lineages of B cells. Although there may be some evidence supporting the existence of the 'so-called' CD5 sister subset (B1b), definitive evidence is not yet available. Particularly, it is presently unclear whether splenic CD5+ B cells share functional and V gene expression characteristics with CD5+ B cells from peritoneal cavity. Indeed, the restricted antibody activity and V gene repertoire expression of these cells have not been found in splenic CD5+ B cells [10, 17, 29, 30].

The human counterpart of the murine Ly1+ B cell is the CD5+ B cell. Ly1 and CD5 molecules have similar primary structures and, in both species, this molecule is also expressed on all T cells [31]. CD5+ B cells account for at least 10% of peripheral normal B cells located in the mantle zone of the follicle, for 2–5% of lymph node B cells [2] and like Ly1-B cells predominate in the fetus and neonate [6, 7]. As is the case for Ly1-B cells, they have been claimed to be mainly involved in polyreactive low-affinity autoantibody secretion [32] for the following reasons. (1) After purification by cytofluorometry, CD5+ B cells infected with Epstein-Barr virus (EBV) under limiting dilution conditions accounted for the vast majority of lymphocytes committed to the production of NAAB [32–34]. (2) Three different groups, including our laboratory, recently unequivocally demonstrated that CD5+ B CLL lymphocytes are frequently involved in the production of these polyreactive NAAB [35–37].

These results and the finding of a high frequency of CD5+ B cells in some autoimmune diseases such as rheumatoid arthritis suggest that CD5+ B cells are involved in the production of NAAB [32–34]. However, the frequency of precursors on polyreactive NAAB in normal healthy subjects is similar to that found in subjects suffering from autoimmune diseases, such as Hashimoto's disease and systemic lupus erythematosus. In these patients, the frequency of B cell precursors of high affinity IgG autoantibodies directed, respectively, against thyroid antigens and DNA, is considerably higher compared to normals, and the latter antibodies appeared to be produced by CD5– B cells [32].

In summary, although there is some evidence that murine Ly1-B and its human counterpart CD5+ B cells may constitute a separate lineage, evidence presently available is not conclusive, and the possibility that CD5 constitutes an activation marker cannot be ruled out since CD5– B cells can be induced to differentiate to CD5+ B cells following treatment with anti-µ and IL-6 [24, 25]. Likewise IL-1 and IL-2, the cytokines that also control the progression of B lymphocytes through the germinal center, are able to downregulate CD5 expression in purified CD5+ B cells [38]. The involvement of CD5+ B cells in the production of NAAB has been demonstrated, but there is some evidence indicating that CD5– B cells may also be involved [20, 26]. Whether CD5+ B cells play an important role in autoimmune diseases remains an unsolved issue.

Progress in the characterization of human B cells has recently been made by associating phenotypic to V gene expression studies in human tonsillar B cells [39, 40]. According to expression of membrane Ig isotypes, CD38, CD77 and CD23, tonsillar B cells can be segregated into three major subsets. Virgin B cells coexpress membrane IgM and IgD, do not express CD38 and may express CD23 (Bm1) or not (Bm2). These cells correspond to mantle zone B cells and are characterized because they express V genes in a configuration close to germline [39, 40]. In contrast, germinal center B cells may express IgM or a switched isotype, do not express IgD, express CD38 and may express CD77 (Bm3) or not (Bm4). Germinal center cells display high levels of somatic mutations [40, 41]. Differentiation towards memory cells is dependent on CD40 signaling, whereas differentiation towards plasma cells is not [42]. Memory B cells are characterized because they have lost membrane IgD and CD38 expression and express in general a switched membrane Ig isotype (may also express IgM) and display a somatic mutation pattern compatible with an antigen-driven process.

V Gene Expression in Chronic Lymphoid Malignancies

It has become apparent during recent years that chronic lymphoid malignancies constitute a heterogeneous group of B and T cell malignancies. The association of morphology with better phenotypic and molecular characterization allowed a better classification of these diseases. The FAB group acknowledged the new findings and published proposals aiming at segregating more objectively the B and T lymphoid leukemias [43, 44]. This classification constitutes an important progress in planning disease therapy, since a number of new and promising treatment modalities have emerged in these diseases, particularly α-interferon and purine nucleoside analogs [45].

Ig variable domains are the combinatorial joining product of V(D)J gene segments. Multisequence comparisons of variable domains have shown that each variable domain contains three regions of extensive sequence variability termed the complementary determining regions (CDRs), and four regions of relative sequence stability termed framework regions [46]. The three light (L) chain CDRs and the three heavy (H) chain CDRs are juxtaposed to form the antigen-binding site of the antibody as classically defined. In turn the framework regions create a scaffold that surrounds, supports, and influences the conformation and structure of the CDRs [47]. In humans, there are 51 functional VH genes distributed into seven families defined because they have a greater than 80% homology within each other. Estimates of the germline VH repertoire showed that the VH1 family was composed of 11 functional members, VH2 of 3, VH3 of 22, VH4 of 11, VH5 of 2, and VH6 and 7 of 1 each [48, 49].

During B cell development, these different VH genes undergo a series of rearrangements with one of the 30 known D gene segments and one of the 6 different JH gene segments. In the case of light chains the rearrangement associates VL (Vκ or Vλ) segments with JL (Jκ or Jλ) gene segments [50, 51]. The human κ locus contains 76 V gene segments including 32 functional genes, 25 pseudogenes and 16 genes with minor defects [52] divided into four different families (VκI to VκIV), and the λ locus appears to contain at least 70 Vλ gene segments belonging to ten different groups [53].

The final product of such a genetic process is the somatically generated genes that encode the two polypeptides (H and L) of the antibody molecules. Thus, in the mature protein the H and L chain CDRs are juxtaposed, with V-encoded CDR1 and 2 regions flanking the V(D)J-derived CDR3 region, thereby forming the center of the antigen-binding site. Sequence diversity in CDR3 is enhanced by the addition of nontemplated nucleotides (N regions) at the splice sites, an activity attributed to TdT. This combinatorial process allows the generation of high numbers of different antibody molecules. However, in B cells, after successful Ig gene rearrangement, a highly specialized process may introduce numerous mutations in the rearranged and expressed Ig V genes [54, 55]. This process that occurs at rates a thousand times higher than normal ($<10^{-3}$/base pair/cell division) and operates only in a subset of B lymphocytes at discrete times during an immune response to antigen allows a generation of high affinity antibodies.

V Gene Expression in CD5+ and CD5– B CLL

B CLL lymphocytes express characteristics low amounts of surface immunoglobulin [23, 56] and CD5 antigen [57–60]. They are resistant to EBV transformation [37, 44], are in a prolonged G0 phase, express high amounts of bcl-2 [61] and display a defective response to different stimuli [62–68]. Despite the presence of many genetic abnormalities, there are no typical chromosomal aberrations or oncogenic abnormalities associated with CLL [45].

Another remarkable characteristic of CLL B cells is their frequent commitment to autoantibody activity [35–37] and the expression of restricted V genes [69–78]. All VH gene families are used and the largest VH3 family is used more frequently, roughly in proportion to its relative size in the genome. In contrast, rearrangements of VH4, VH5 and VH6 family members occur more frequently than expected from their respective size in the genome [28, 73–78].

Interestingly, developmentally restricted Ig genes, which are often associated with anti-idiotype cross-reactivity, are preferentially used in a germline configuration [70, 71]. Different studies on Ig gene expression in B CLL have shown a nonrandom use of V regions and the frequent expression of V genes in a germinal configuration. Data from 75 CLL cases where the complete gene sequence was identified [78] showed the expression of 27 different genes. However, genes V1-69 (51P1), 4-34 (4-21), 4-39 (4-18) and V5-52 (VH5-251) accounted for 37 of the 75 cases. The pattern of somatic mutations is heterogeneous, half of the cases displaying an unmutated germinal pattern, while the other half contained a significant amount of mutations, some of which may correspond to polymorphisms inherited in the germline DNA. This differential pattern of mutations addresses the question as to whether CLL B cell malignant hits could occur at different steps of B cell ontogeny. In addition, in contrast to other B cell malignancies there is a lack of intraclonal diversity [28].

The rare cases expressing IgG isotype tend to use more frequently mutated VH genes with evidence of antigen selection in some cases [73], although the two cases using the V4-39 gene, as it occurs for IgM-expressing CLLs, employed this gene in a germline configuration. More recently, the same group showed that IgM+ B cells, which are precursors of the leukemic B cells, exist in increased numbers in the blood of most patients with IgG+ B CLL and that these cells may differentiate, accumulate V gene mutations, and undergo isotype switching in vivo [79]. Interestingly, in IgM-expressing CLL, IgG and IgA transcripts were also found. cDNA cloning and sequencing showed that the VDJ segments associated with γ and α heavy chain transcripts were identical to those from mu transcripts, thus showing that B lymphocytes giving rise to CLL cells have undergone isotype switching in vivo. Comparison and alignment of these sequences to corresponding germline genes showed little or no somatic mutations [80, 81]. Thomsett et al. [82] analyzed VH gene expression in CD5+ B CLL correlating the results to the cytogenetic abnormalities. Results showed that the cases with chromosome 13 abnormalities used mutated VH genes, whereas mutations were infrequently observed in the case of patients displaying trisomy 12.

In mice and humans, B cells that arise early in ontogeny are enriched for CD5 expression [6, 7]. The ability to respond to specific antigens and expression of V genes are developmentally controlled in both species [83, 84]. In addition to differences in the VH repertoire, there are significant differences in the composition, sequence and length distribution of the H chain CDR3 intervals in cord blood when compared with those identified in the fetus [78].

Fetal transcripts are enriched in DHQ52, the shortest of the human DH gene segments and frequently use JH3 and 4 segments, whereas cord blood transcripts are enriched for gene segments of the longer DXP family and frequently employ the larger JH5 and JH6 segments, as well as JH4 and more rarely JH3. In addition, cord blood transcripts contain more N region additions than fetal transcripts. As a consequence of enhanced N additions and use of longer DH and JH gene segments, cord blood CDR3 sequences have an average length of 17 codons, which is 6 codons longer than the average fetal CDR3 length of 11 codons. Since early results showed an overexpression of developmentally restricted VH genes [70, 71] and CD5+ B cells have been reported to predominate during early ontogeny [6, 7], the possibility exists that CLL could correspond to the expansion of an immature B cell, expressing a repertoire of developmentally restricted V genes. The study of CDR3 regions can serve as a marker for populations of V domains derived from fetal versus mature B cells. This study carried out on 50 different H chain transcripts showed a pattern compatible with mature B cells [78].

The exact position of the CD5 antigen during B cell ontogeny is still unclear. To obtain more information on this issue, we addressed the question as to whether B cells proliferating in CD5– B CLL are derived as is the case for CD5+ B CLL from the same naive pregerminal low mutated B cell pool, or whether they could be derived from highly mutated germinal center-derived memory B cells.

CD5– B CLLs represent less than 5% of B CLLs. When compared with CD5+ B CLLs, more cases have advanced disease, splenomegaly, and a cytological mixed CLL pattern according to the French-American-British (FAB) classification [85]. In addition, the CD23 expression is frequently absent, whereas FMC7 positivity and expression of high amounts of sIg are more frequently observed than in CD5+ B CLLs [86]. Thus, CD5– B CLL seems to be intermediate between classical CLL and prolymphocytic leukemia (PLL) [85]. We analyzed the VH genes used in 11 cases of CD5– B CLL for the presence of somatic mutations. The results showed no differences in terms of VH family usage, but a higher mutation pattern, following a random distribution, was observed when comparing these results to those described in CD5+ B CLL [87]. In a single case of CD5– B CLL [72], a tendency to express genes displaying a higher number of somatic mutations was also reported. These results appeared, however, to be related to the membrane Ig phenotype, since less mutations were observed in membrane μδ expressing CLLs, when compared to forms exclusively expressing membrane μ [87]. Interestingly, a recent report in normal B cells showed that B cells expressing the μδ phenotype displayed lower somatic mutation rates than μ and γ expressing

B cells [88]. In addition, similar results were found in 5 cases of splenic lymphoma with villous lymphocytes [89]. This differential pattern of somatic mutations among variable domains observed among CLL patients could provide information concerning the particular stage of development in which malignant transformation has occurred and could suggest that CLL may be a heterogeneous disorder that could involve naive cells at different stages of development ($\mu\delta$, μ or even γ isotype expression). However, this is not a constant phenomenon, since one case expressing exclusively μ at the membrane displayed a V1-69 gene in a germline configuration and one case expressing membrane $\mu\delta$ showed a homology of 95.4% with its closest germinal counterpart. Furthermore, taking into account that this difference was observed in a limited series of patients, it needs to be confirmed in a larger number of patients.

VH Gene Expression in Mantle Cell Lymphoma

Mantle cell lymphoma (MCL) is characterized histologically by neoplastic expansion of the mantle zone surrounding lymph node germinal centers [90, 91]. Immunophenotyping by flow cytometry and immunocytochemistry have demonstrated that the malignant lymphocytes of MCL characteristically express high density surface $\mu\delta$, CD19, CD20, CD22, and CD5. The lack of expression of CD23 is useful in distinguishing MCL from CLL in which the antigen density of CD20 and surface Ig is typically much lower than the expression of these molecules on MCL cells [90, 92]. A cytogenetic analysis of MCL has revealed a characteristic t(11;14) translocation involving the Ig heavy chain gene on chromosome 14 and the bcl-1 oncogene on chromosome 11 [93–95]. To determine whether MCL are related to naive pregerminal center B cells (expressing nonmutated rearranged VH genes) or to germinal center-derived B cells (expressing mutated rearranged VH genes), Hummel et al. [96] sequenced VH genes used in six MCLs and analyzed them for the presence of somatic mutations. The VH region sequences of these cases showed no or very little somatic mutations, indicating that MCL cells may derive from naive pregerminal center B cells. However, Oscier et al. [97] reported a VH gene analysis of 8 MCL cases, showing heterogeneity in the incidence of somatic mutation events with 2/8 unmutated but 6/8 with high levels of mutation. As observed in B CLL, no intraclonal diversity could be found. Overall, the results from these reports appear to reach opposite conclusions, and more studies are needed to answer this question.

VH Gene Expression in Splenic Lymphoma with Villous Lymphocytes

Splenic lymphoma with villous lymphocytes (SLVL) is a low grade B cell lymphoma that usually presents with splenomegaly in the absence of lymph node enlargement [98]. Approximately 70% of cases have an abnormal karyotype with a preponderance of abnormalities involving chromosome 11q13, 7q, 17q and 2p11. Fifteen percent of patients have a characteristic t(11;14)(q13;q32), though the rearrangements of the bcl-1 locus in SLVL appear diverse and may be distinct from those of MCL [99]. Analysis of the nucleotide sequences of VH region used in five typical cases of SLVL showed somatic hypermutation from germline sequences in all cases, indicating that the cell of origin has been exposed to the hypermutation mechanism. However no clonal diversity was detectable, demonstrating that the tumor cell does not accumulate further mutations. The distribution of mutations leading to amino acid replacement differed among the cases, with 3 out of the 5 cases showing a pattern compatible with an antigen-driven process. It is of note that CD5 expression did not appear to be related to the mutational pattern and mutations were lower in the $\mu\delta$ expressing cases [100].

VH Gene Expression in PLL

PLL is a chronic lymphoproliferative disorder characterized by prominent splenomegaly, prolymphocytes accounting more than 55% of circulating lymphocytes, and short-term survival [43, 101]. The majority of PLLs are from the B lineage origin and express high-density monotypic surface membrane Ig, usually IgM with or without IgD, and the CD19, CD20 and CD22 cell markers. In contrast to B CLL, they often express FMC7, high density surface membrane Ig and in about half of the cases CD5 molecule, but rarely CD23 [102–104]. In order to better define the nature of the cellular origin in PLL, we analyzed VH genes in 11 cases of de novo PLL. Leukemic cells expressed a skewed repertoire characterized by the predominant use of VH3 family members (73%) with a preferential utilization of the V3-23 gene (50% of the VH3 genes used). In most cases the VH genes expressed diverged from their putative germline counterpart with a mutation rate greater than 5%. The type and distribution of these mutations were compatible in at least 3 of the cases studied with an antigen-driven process. There was no evidence of intraclonal heterogeneity, suggesting that the mutation mechanism was no longer operational in the tumor cells. These results suggest that B PLL cells probably represent expansion of postgerminal center cells which, at least in some cases, have undergone an antigen-driven process [105].

Conclusion

Although there is some evidence that murine Ly1-B and its human counter-part CD5+ B (B1a) and the CD5– B (B1b) sister cells may constitute a separate lineage from conventional (B2) B cells, evidence presently available is not conclu-sive, and the possibility that CD5 constitutes an activation marker cannot be ruled out. In mice, where the evidence is more convincing, it is presently unclear whether splenic CD5+ B cells share functional and V gene expression characteris-tics with CD5+ B cells from the peritoneal cavity. Indeed, the restricted antibody activity and V gene repertoire expression of these cells have not been found in splenic CD5+ B cells [10, 17, 29, 30]. The involvement of CD5+ B cells in the production of NAAB has been demonstrated, but there is some evidence indicat-ing that CD5– B cells may also be involved [20, 26]. Whether CD5+ B cells play an important role in autoimmune diseases and whether they express a different set of V genes remains an unsolved issue. In humans, important progress has been made in the identification of B cell subsets, which can presently be characterized according to the expression of different phenotypic markers. Hence, virgin naive B cells, which display a configuration of V genes close to germline, express mem-brane μδ and do not express CD38. Germinal center cells characterized by high levels of mutations do not express δ, express CD38 and frequently express a switched membrane Ig. Finally, memory B cells fail to express δ and CD38, fre-quently express a switched membrane Ig and display a characteristic antigen-driven mutation pattern.

The composition of Ig loci reflects the developmental stage of B cells. Analy-ses of VH genes expressed in normal B cells and during B cell malignancies can be added to the phenotypic, karyotypic and functional studies, to gain more insight into B cell differentiation. When studying VH gene expression in B cell malignan-cies throughout B cell development, we propose a molecular classification based on VH usage and their mutation pattern which help designing the origin of the B cell. In normal pre-B cells and particularly in acute lymphoblastic leukemia pre-B cells, as expected, VH genes are used in their germline configuration [106, 107]. In contrast, follicular lymphomas [108, 109], diffuse large cell lymphomas [110], multiple myelomas [111, 112] and mucosa-associated lymphoid tissue lympho-mas [113, 114] express mutated VH genes with or without intraclonal diversity. The fact that mutations and replacements predominate in CDRs suggests that these clones have undergone an antigen-driven process. In CLL and MCL analy-ses of VH expression may suggest that these diseases are heterogeneous and that the malignant hit(s) could occur at different stages of B cell development. Although the expression of CD5 is characteristic of mantle zone cells and could be associated with a low mutational rate observed in these B cell malignancies, our results comparing CD5+ and CD5– B CLL and B PLL do not demonstrate impor-

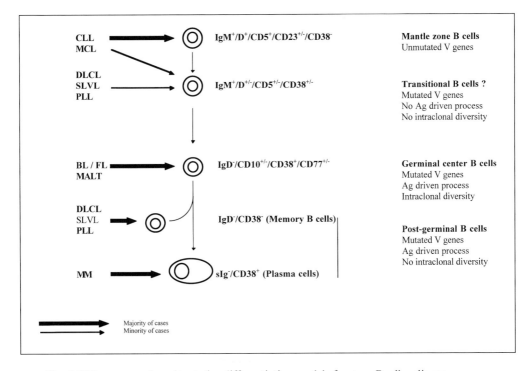

Fig. 1. VH gene usage-based tentative differentiation model of mature B cell malignancies. CLL and MCL expressing generally CD5 antigen and unmutated V genes correspond to virgin B cells. However, in some cases, particularly in CD5– B CLL cases as well as some cases of PLL and SLVL, VH genes are slightly mutated. These 'transitional' B cells include B cells which cannot be allocated according to the phenotype or the V gene usage to mantle zone or germinal center cells. In the majority of diffuse large cell lymphoma (DLCL), PLL and SLVL cases, VH genes display a mutated pattern without intraclonal diversity. Burkitt lymphoma (BL), follicular lymphoma (FL), and mucosa-associated lymphoid tissue (MALT) lymphoma cells use VH-mutated V genes which displayed intraclonal heterogeneity. MM = Multiple myelomas.

tant differences in the mutational pattern related to CD5 expression. In agreement with the new proposal they tend to show that the level of mutations observed could be related to the Ig membrane isotype (more mutations in μ-expressing cases when compared to those simultaneously expressing μδ). According to the new phenotypic distinction of B cells, CLL and MCL cases expressing CD5 antigen and membrane μδ, with little or no somatic mutation, could correspond to expansion of the virgin naive B cell. In contrast, follicular lymphomas which fail to express membrane δ and express CD38 and a high mutational pattern with intraclonal diversity probably correspond to the expansion of germinal center B cells. Myeloma cells exhibit a genotypic VH pattern close to postgerminal memory B cells. Taken together, these results can help to propose a hypothetical classification of B cell malignancies based on immunophenotypic and molecular studies (fig. 1). Although other B cell disorders such as PLL, SLVL, CD5– B CLL and some cases of MCL with a high mutation rate can be included in this tentative model, further work is necessary to substantiate this hypothesis.

Acknowledgments

We would like to thank Ms. S. Demolliere and Ms. R.A. Bouyssié for secretarial assistance.

References

1   Herzenberg LA, Stall AM, Lalor PA, Sidman C, Mosse WA, Parly DR, Herzenberg LA: The Ly1-B cell lineage. Immunol Rev 1986;93:81.
2   Hardy R, Hayakawa K: Development and physiology of Ly-1 B and its human homolog, Leu-1B. Immunol Rev 1986;93:53.
3   Cantor H, Boyse EA: Functional subclasses of T lymphocytes bearing different Ly antigens. I. The generation of functionally distinct T-cell subclasses in a differentiation process independent of antigen. J Exp Med 1975;141:1376.
4   Manohar V, Brown E, Leiserson WM, Chused TM: Expression of Ly-1 by a subset of B lymphocytes. J Immunol 1982;129:532.
5   Hayakawa K, Hardy RR, Parks DR: The Ly-1B cell subpopulation in normal immunodefective and autoimmune mice. J Exp Med 1983;157:202.
6   Bofil M, Janossy G, Janossa M, Burford GD, Seymour GJ, Wernet P, Kelemen E: Human B cell development H. Subpopulations in the human fetus. J Immunol 1985;134:1531.
7   Antin JH, Emerson SP, Martin P, Gaddol N, Adult KA: Leu 1 (CD5) B cells, a major lymphoid subpopulation in human fetal spleen: Phenotypic and functional studies. Immunology 1986;136: 505.
8   Hayakawa K, Hardy RR, Herzenberg LA, Herzenberg LA: Progenitors for Ly-1 B cells are distinct from progenitors for other B cells. J Exp Med 1985;161:1554.
9   Hayakawa K, Hardy RR, Stall AM, Herzenberg LA, Herzenberg LA: Immunoglobulin bearing B cells reconstitute and maintain the murine Ly-1 B cell lineage. Eur J Immunol 1986;16:1313.
10 Pennel CA, Arnold LW, Haughton G, Clarke SH: Restricted Ig variable region gene expression among Ly-1 B cell lymphomas. J Immunol 1988;141:2788.
11 Gu H, Forster I, Rajewsky K: Sequence homologies, N sequence insertion and JH gene utilization in VHDJH joining: Implications for the joining mechanism and the ontogenetic timing of Ly1 B cell and B-CLL progenitor generation. EMBO J 1990;9:2133.
12 Hayakawa K, Hardy RR, Honda M, Herzenberg LA, Steinberg AD, Herzenberg LA: Ly-1 B cells: Functionally distinct lymphocytes that secrete IgM autoantibodies. Proc Natl Acad Sci USA 1984; 81:2494.
13 Sidman CL, Shultz LD, Hardy RR, Hayakawa K, Herzenberg LA: Production of immunoglobulin isotypes by Ly-1+ B cells in viable motheaten and normal mice. Science 1986;232:1423.
14 Dighiero G, Lymberi P, Holmberg D, Lundquist I, Coutinho A, Avrameas S: High frequency of natural autoantibodies in normal newborn mice. J Immunol 1985;134:765.
15 Dighiero G, Lim A, Poncet P, Kaushik A, Ge XR, Mazié JC: Age-related natural antibody specificities among hybridoma clones originating from NZB spleen. Immunology 1987;62:341.

16 Bussard AE, Vinit MA, Pages JM: Immunochemical characterization of the autoantibodies produced by mouse peritoneal cells in culture. Immunochemistry 1976;14:1.

17 Tornberg UC, Holmberg D: B-1a and B-2 B cells display unique VHDJH repertoires formed at different stages of ontogeny and under different selection pressures. EMBO J 1995;14:1680.

18 Theofilopoulos AN, Dixon FJ: Murine models of systemic lupus erythematosus. Adv Immunol 1985;37:269.

19 Schwartz RS, Datta SK: Autoimmunity and autoimmune diseases; in Paul WE (ed): Fundamental Immunology, ed 2. New York, Raven Press, 1989.

20 Dighiero G, Poncet P, Rouyre S, Mazié JC: New-born Xid mice carry the genetic information for the production of natural autoantibodies. J Immunol 1986;136:4000.

21 Kaushik A, Lim A, Poncet P, Ge XR, Dighiero G: Comparative analysis of natural antibody specificities among hybridomas originating from spleen and peritoneal cavity of adult NZB and BALB/c mice. Scand J Immunol 1988;27:461.

22 Kaushik A, Mayer R, Fidanza V, Zaghouani H, Lim A, Bona C, Dighiero G: Ly1 and V-gene expression among hybridomas secreting natural autoantibody. J Autoimmun 1990;3:687.

23 Ternynck T, Dighiero G, Follezou JY, Binet JL: Comparison of normal and CLL lymphocytes surface Ig determinants using peroxidase-labeled antibodies. I. Detection and quantification of light chain determinants. Blood 1974;43:789.

24 Yingzi C, Rabin E, Wortis HH: Treatment of murine CD5– B cells with anti-Ig, but no LPS, induces surface CD5: Two B-cell activation pathways. Int Immunol 1990;3:467.

25 Wortis HH, Teutsch M, Higer M, Zheng J, Parker DC: B-cell activation by crosslinking of surface IgM or ligation of CD40 involves alternative signal pathways and results in different B-cell phenotypes. Proc Natl Acad Sci USA 1995;92:3348–3352.

26 Dighiero G, Hart S, Lim A, Borche L, Levy R, Miller RA: Autoantibody activity of immunoglobulins isolated from B-cell follicular lymphomas. Blood 1991;78:581.

27 Kantor AB: The development and repertoire of B-1 cells (CD5 B cells). Immunol Today 1991;12: 389.

28 Kipps TJ, Carson DA: Autoantibodies in chronic lymphocytic leukemia and related systemic autoimmune diseases. Blood 1995;81:2475.

29 Poncet P, Reininger L, Freitas A, Holmberg D, Dighiero G, Coutinho A: Expression of VH11-gene family in hybridoma collections from peritoneum and spleen. Differential correlation with BrMRBC reactivity. Res Immunol 1989;140:255.

30 Dighiero G, Lim A, Lembezat MP, Kaushik A, Andrade L, Freitas A: Comparative usage of VH gene family usage by newborn Xid and non-Xid mice, newborn NZB and adult NZB and by splenic and peritoneal cavity B cell compartments. Eur J Immunol 1989;18:1979.

31 Huang HJ, Jones NH, Strominger JL: Molecular cloning of Ly-1, a membrane glycoprotein of mouse T lymphocytes and a subset of B cells: Molecular homology to its human counterpart Leu-1/T1 (CD5). Proc Natl Acad Sci USA 1987;84:204.

32 Casali P, Notkins AL: Probing the human B-cell repertoire with EBV: Polyreactive and CD5+ B lymphocytes. Annu Rev Immunol 1989;7:513.

33 Hardy RR, Hayakawa K, Shimizu M, Yamasaki K, Kishimoto T: Rheumatoid factor secretion from human Leu-1+ B cells. Science 1987;236:81.

34 Casali P, Burastero SE, Nakamura M, Inghirami G, Notkins AL: Human lymphocytes making rheumatoid factors and antibodies to single stranded DNA belong to the Leu-1+ B cell subset. Science 1987;236:77.

35 Bröker BM, Klajman A, Youinou P, Jouquan J, Worman CP, Murphy J, Mackenzie L, Quartey-Papafio R, Blaschek M, Collins P, Lal S, Lydyard PM: Chronic lymphocytic leukemic (CLL) cells secrete multispecific autoantibodies. J Autoimmun 1988;1:469.

36 Sthoeger ZM, Wakai M, Tse DB, Vinciguerra VP, Allen SL, Budman DR, Lichtman SM, Schulman P, Weiselberg LR, Chiorazzi N: Production of autoantibodies by CD5-expressing B lymphocytes from patients with chronic lymphocytic leukemia. J Exp Med 1989;169:255.

37 Borche L, Lim A, Binet JL, Dighiero G: Evidence that chronic lymphocytic leukemia B lymphocytes are frequently committed to productions of natural autoantibodies. Blood 1990;76:562.

38   Caligaris-Cappio F, Riva M, Tesio L, Schena M, Gaidano GL, Bergui L: Human normal CD5+ B lymphocytes can be induced to differentiate to CD5– B lymphocytes with germinal center cell features. Blood 1989;73:1259.

39   Küppers R, Zhao M, Hansmann ML, Rajewsky K: Tracing B cell development in human germline centres by molecular analysis of single cells from histological sections. EMBO J 1993;12:4955.

40   Pascual V, Liu YJ, Magalski A, de Bouteiller O, Banchereau J, Capra JD: Analysis of somatic mutation in five B cell subsets of human tonsil. J Exp Med 1994;180:329–339.

41   Liu YJ, de Bouteiller O, Arpin C, Durand I, Banchereau J: Five human mature B cell subsets. Adv Exp Med Biol 1994;355:289–296.

42   Arpin C, Dechanet J, Van Kooten C, Merville P, Grouard G, Briere F, Banchereau J, Liu YJ: Generation of memory B cells and plasma cells in vitro. Science 1995;268:720.

43   Bennett JM, Catovsky D, Daniel MT, Flandrin G, Galton DAG, Gralnick HR, Sultan C: Proposals for the classification of chronic (mature) B and T lymphoid leukemias. J Clin Pathol 1989;42:567.

44   Catovsky D: Diagnosis and treatment of CLL variants; in Cheson BD (ed): Chronic Lymphocytic Leukemia. Scientific Advances and Clinical Developments. New York, Dekker, 1993, p 369.

45   Dighiero G, Travade P, Chevret S, Fenaux P, Chastang C, Binet JL: The French Cooperative Group on CLL: B-cell chronic lymphocytic leukemia. Present status and future directions. Blood 1991;78: 1901.

46   Kabat EA, Wu TT, Perry HM, Gottesman KS, Foeller C: Sequences of Proteins of Immunological Interest. Bethesda, US Department of Health and Human Services, 1991.

47   Kirkham PM, Schroeder HW: Antibody structure and the evolution of immunoglobulin V gene segments. Semin Immunol 1994;6:347.

48   Matsuda F, Shin EK, Nagaoka H, Matsumara R, Haino M, Fukita Y, Taka-ishi S, Imai T, Riley JH, Anand R, Soeda E, Honjo T: Structure and physical map of 64 variables segments in the 3′ 0.8-megabase region of the human immunoglobulin heavy-chain locus. Nature Genet 1993;3:88.

49   Tomlinson IM, Walter G, Marks JD, Llewelyn MB, Winter G: The repertoire of human germline VH segments reveals about fifty groups of VH segments with different hypervariable loops. J Mol Biol 1992;227:776.

50   Tonegawa S: Somatic generation of antibody diversity. Nature 1983;302:575.

51   Pascual V, Capra JD: Human immunoglobulin heavy-chain variable region genes: Organization, polymorphism and expression. Adv Immunol 1991;49:1.

52   Klein R, Jaenichen R, Zachau HG: Expressed human immunoglobulin κ genes and their hypermutation. Eur J Immunol 1993;23:3248–3271.

53   Frippiat JP, Lefranc MP: Genomic organization of 34 kb of the human immunoglobulin lambda locus (IGLV): Restriction map and sequences of new VλIII genes. Mol Immunol 1994;31:657–670.

54   McKean D, Huppi K, Bell M, Staudt L, Gerhard W, Weigert M: Generation of antibody diversity in the immune response of BALB/c mice to influenza virus hemagglutinin. Proc Natl Acad Sci USA 1984;81:3180.

55   Griffiths GM, Berek C, Kaartinen M, Milstein C: Somatic mutation and the maturation of the immune response to 2-phenyl oxazzolone. Nature 1984;312:271.

56   Dighiero G, Bodega E, Mayzner R, Binet JL: Individual cell-by-cell quantitation of lymphocyte surface membrane Ig in normal and CLL lymphocytes and during ontogeny of mouse B lymphocytes by immunoperoxidase assay. Blood 1980;55:93.

57   Boumsell L, Bernard A, Lepage V: Some chronic lymphocytic leukemia cells bearing surface immunoglobulins share determinants with T cells. Eur J Immunol 1978;8:900.

58   Royston I, Majda JA, Baird SM, Mirserve BE, Griffiths EC: Human T-cell antigens defined by monoclonal antibodies: The 65000 dalton antigen of immunoglobulin. J Immunol 1980;125:725.

59   Caligaris-Cappio E, Gobbi M, Bofill M, Janossy G: Infrequent normal B lymphocytes express features of B-chronic lymphocytic leukemia. J Exp Med 1985;155:623.

60   Caligaris-Cappio F, Janossy G: Surface markers in chronic lymphoid leukemias of B cell type. Semin Hematol 1985;22:1.

61   Gottardi D, Alfarano A, De Leo AM, Stacchini A, Bergui L, Caligaris-Cappio F: Defective apoptosis due to Bcl-2 overexpression may explain why B-CLL cells accumulate in GO. Curr Top Microbiol Immunol 1995;194:307–312.

62 Hivroz C, Grillot-Courvalin C, Brouet JC, Seligmann M: Heterogeneity of responsiveness of chronic lymphocytic leukemic B cells to B cell growth factor or interleukin 2. Eur J Immunol 1986; 16:1001.

63 Karray S, DeFrance T, Merle-Béral H, Bancherau J, Debré P, Galanaud P: Interleukin 4 counteracts the interleukin 2-induced proliferation of monoclonal B cells. J Exp Med 1988;168:85.

64 Karray S, Merle-Béral H, Vazquez A, Gérard JP, Debré P, Galanaud P: Functional heterogeneity of B-CLL lymphocytes: Dissociated responsiveness to growth factors and distinct requirements for a first activation signal. Blood 1987;70:1105.

65 Fluckiger AC, Briere F, Zurawski G, Bridon JM, Bancherau J: IL-13 has only a subset of IL-4-like activities on B chronic lymphocytic leukaemia cells. Immunology 1994;83:397.

66 Fluckiger AC, Durand I, Bancherau J: Interleukin 10 induces apoptotic cell death of B-chronic lymphocytic leukemia cells. J Exp Med 1994;179:91.

67 Fluckiger AC, Garrone P, Durand I, Galizzi JP, Bancherau J: Interleukin 10 (IL-10) upregulates functional high affinity IL-2 receptors on normal and leukemic B lymphocytes. J Exp Med 1993; 178:1473.

68 Michel F, Merle-Béral H, Legac E, Michel A, Debré P, Bismuth G: Defective calcium response in B-chronic lymphocytic leukemia cells. Alteration of early protein tyrosine phosphorylation and of the mechanism responsible for cell calcium influx. J Immunol 1993;150:3624–3633.

69 Shen A, Humphries C, Tucker P, Blattner F: Human heavy-chain variable region gene family nonrandomly rearranged in familial chronic lymphocytic leukemia. Proc Natl Acad Sci USA 1987;84: 8563.

70 Kipps TJ, Tomhave E, Chen PP, Carson DA: Autoantibody associated K light chain variable region gene expressed in chronic lymphocytic leukemia with little or no somatic mutation, implications for etiology and immunotherapy. J Exp Med 1988;167:840.

71 Kipps TJ, Tomhave E, Pratt LF, Duffy S, Chen PP, Carson DA: Developmentally restricted immunogloublin heavy chain variable region gene expressed at high frequency in chronic lymphocytic leukemia. Proc Natl Acad Sci USA 1989;86:5913.

72 Roudier J, Silverman GJ, Chen PP, Carson DA, Kipps TJ: Intraclonal diversity in the VH genes expressed by CD5– chronic lymphocytic leukemia-producing pathologic IgM rheumatoid factors. J Immunol 1990;144:1526.

73 Logtenberg T, Schutte MEM, Inghirami G, Berman JE, Gmelig-Meyling FHJ, Insel RA, Knowles DM, Alt FW: Immunoglobulin VH gene expression in human B cell lines and tumors: Biased VH expression in chronic lymphocytic leukemia. Int Immunol 1989;1:362.

74 Deane M, Norton JD: Immunoglobulin heavy chain variable region family usage is independent of tumor cell phenotype in human B lineage leukemias. Eur J Immunol 1990;20:2209.

75 Mayer R, Logtenberg T, Strauchen J, Dimitriu-Bona A, Mayer L, Mechanic S, Chiorazzi N, Borche L, Dighiero G, Mannheimer-Lory A, Diamond B, Alt FW, Bona C: CD5 and immunoglobulin V gene expression in B-cell lymphomas and chronic lymphocytic leukemia. Blood 1990;75:1518.

76 Hashimoto S, Wakai M, Silver J, Chiorazzi N: Biased usage of variable and constant region genes by IgG+, CD5+ human leukemic B cells. Ann NY Acad Sci 1992;651:477.

77 Pritsch O, Magnac C, Dumas G, Egile C, Dighiero G: V gene usage by seven hybrids derived from CD5+ B-CLL and displaying autoantibody activity. Blood 1993;151:3103.

78 Schroeder HW, Dighiero G: The pathogenesis of chronic lymphocytic leukemia: Analysis of the antibody repertoire. Immunol Today 1994;15:288.

79 Hashimoto S, Dono M, Wakai M, Allen SL, Lichtman SM, Schulman P, Vinciguerra VP, Ferrarini M, Silver J, Chiorazzi N: Somatic diversification and selection of immunoglobulin heavy and light chain variable region genes in IgG+ CD5+ chronic lymphocytic leukemia B. J Exp Med 1995;181: 1507–1517.

80 Dono M, Hashimoto S, Ferrarini M, Chiorazzi N: In vivo isotype class switching in CD5+ chronic lymphocytic leukemia B cells. Ann NY Acad Sci 1995;764:478–481.

81 Malisan F, Fluckiger AC, Ho S, Guret C, Bancherau J, Martinez-Valdez H: B chronic lymphocytic leukemias can undergo isotype switching in vivo and can be induced to differentiate and switch in vitro. Blood 1996;87:717–724.

82 Thomsett A, Zhu D, Stevenson F: Differential rates of somatic hypermutation in VH genes among subsets of chronic lymphocytic leukemia defined by chromosomal abnormalities. Blood 1995; 86(suppl 1):840a.

83 Yancopoulos GD, Desiderio SV, Paskind M, Kearney JF, Baltimore D, Alt F: Preferential utilization of the most JH-proximal VH gene segments in pre-B cell lines. Nature 1984;311:727.

84 Schroeder HW, Hilson JL, Perlmutter RM: Early restriction of the human antibody repertoire. Science 1987;238:791.

85 Salomon-Nguyen F, Valensi F, Merle-Béral H, Flandrin G: A scoring system for the classification of CD5-B CLL versus CD5+ B CLL and B PLL. Leukemia and lymphoma. Leuk Lymphoma 1995;16: 445.

86 Geisler CH, Larsen JK, Hansen NE, Hansen MM, Christensen BE, Lund B, Nielsen H, Plesner T, Thorling K, Andersen PK: Prognostic importance of flow cytometric immunophenotyping of 540 consecutive patients with B-cell chronic lymphocytic leukemia. Blood 1991;78:1795.

87 Maloum K, Davi F, Magnac C, Pritsch O, McIntyre E, Valensi F, Binet JL, Merle-Béral H, Dighiero G: Analysis of VH gene expression in CD5+ and CD5-negative B-cell chronic lymphocytic leukemia. Blood 1995;86:3883–3890.

88 Klein U, Küppers R, Rajewsky K: Human IgM + IgD + B cells, the major B cell subset in the peripheral blood express VH genes with no or little somatic mutation throughout life. Eur J Immunol 1993;23:3272.

90 Banks PM, Chan J, Cleary ML, et al: Mantle cell lymphoma: A proposal for unification of morphologic and molecular data. Am J Surg Pathol 1992;16:637–640.

91 Harris NL, Jaffe ES, Stein H, et al: A revised European-American classification of lymphoid neoplasms: A proposal from the international lymphoma study group. Blood 1994;84:1361–1392.

92 Zukerberg L, Medeiros L, Ferry J, Harris N: Diffuse low grade B cell lymphomas: Four clinically distinct subtypes defined by a combination of morphology and immunophenotypic features. Am J Clin Pathol 1993;100:373–385.

93 Rimokh R, Berger F, Delsol G, et al: Detection of the chromosomal translocation t(11:14) by polymerase chain reaction in mantle cell lymphomas. Blood 1994;83:1871–1875.

94 Mobt RJ, Meeker TC, Wittwer CT, et al: Antigen expression and polymerase chain reaction amplification of mantle cell lymphomas. Blood 1994;83:1626–1631.

95 De Boer Carla J, Shuuring ED, Dreif E, et al: Cyclin D1 protein analysis in the diagnosis of MCL. Blood 1995;86:2715–2723.

96 Hummel M, Tamaru JI, Kalvelage B, Stein H: Mantle cell (previously centrocytic) lymphomas express V_H genes with no or very little somatic mutations like the physiologic cells of the follicle mantle. Blood 1994;84:403.

97 Oscier DG, Matutes E, Zhu D, Stevenson F: Chronic lymphoproliferative disorders associated with the t(11;14) translocation have VH genes with a widely variable incidence of somatic hypermutation. Blood 1995;86(suppl 1):819a.

98 Melo JV, Hedge V, Parreira A, Thompson I, Lampert IA, Catovsky D: Splenic B-cell lymphoma with circulating villous lymphocytes: Differential diagnosis of B-cell leukemia with large spleens. J Clin Pathol 1987;40:642.

99 Oscier DG, Matutes E, Gardiner A, Glide S, Mould S, Brito-Babapulle V, Ellis J, Catovsky D: Cytogenetic studies in splenic lymphoma with villous lymphocytes. Br J Haematol 1993;85:487.

100 Zhu D, Oscier DG, Stevenson K: Splenic lymphoma with villous lymphocytes involves B cells with extensively mutated Ig heavy chain variable region genes. Blood 1995;85:1603.

101 Galton DAG, Goldman JM, Wiltshaw E, Catovsky D, Henry K, Goldenberg GJ: Prolymphocytic leukemia. Br J Haematol 1974;27:7.

102 Dighiero G, Follezou JY, Roisin JP, Ternynck T, Binet JL: Comparison of normal and chronic lymphocytic leukemia lymphocyte surface Ig determinants using peroxidase-labeled antibodies. II. Quantification of light chain determinants in atypical lymphocytic leukemia. Blood 1976;48:559.

103 Melo JV, Catovsky D, Galton DAG: The relationship between chronic lymphocytic leukemia and prolymphocytic leukemia. I. Clinical and laboratory features of 300 patients and characterization of an intermediate group. Br J Haematol 1986;63:377.

104 Melo JV, Catovsky D, Galton DAG: The relationship between chronic lymphocytic leukemia and prolymphocytic leukemia. Part II. Br J Haematol 1986;64:77.

105 Davi F, Maloum K, Michel A, Pritsch O, Magnac C, McIntyre E, Salomon-Nguyen F, Binet JL, Dighiero G, Merle-Béral H: Frequent somatic mutations in the VH genes expressed in prolympho-cytic leukemia. Blood 1996;88:3953–3961.

106 Deane M, Baker BW, Norton JD: Immunoglobulin VH4 usage in B lymphoid leukemias. Br J Haematol 1993;84:242–249.

107 Maloum K, Magnac C, Pritsh O, Binet JL, Merle-Béral H, Dighiero G: Skewed rearrangement of the VH4-21 gene during PRE-B acute lymphoblastic leukemia. Leuk Lymphoma 1995;17:435–441.

108 Bahler DW, Campbell MJ, Hart S, Miller RA, Levy S, Levy R: IgVH gene expression among human follicular lymphomas. Blood 1991;78:1561.

109 Zelenetz AD, Chen TT, Levy R: Clonal expansion in FL occurs subsequent to antigenic selection. J Exp Med 1992;176:1137.

110 Hsu FJ, Levy R: Preferential use of the VH4 gene family by diffuse large cell lymphoma. Blood 1995;86:3072–3082.

111 Bakkus MHC, Heirman C, Van Riet I, Van Camp B, Thielemans K: Evidence that multiple myelo-ma Ig heavy chain VDJ genes contain somatic mutations but show no intraclonal variation. Blood 1992;80:2326.

112 Sahoto SS, Leo R, Hamblin TJ, Stevenson FK: Ig Vh gene mutational patterns indicate different tumor cell status in human myeloma and monoclonal gammopathy of undetermined significance. Blood 1996;87:746–755.

113 Du MQ, Diss TC, Xu CF, Peng HZ, Isaacson PG, Pan LX: Somatic mutations and intraclonal variations in MALT lymphomas immunoglobulin genes. Blood 1995;86(suppl 1):181a.

114 Miklos JA, Swerdlow SH, Bahler DW: Analysis of immunoglobulin VH genes used by low grade salivary gland lymphomas of the mucosa associated lymphoid tissue (MALT) type. Blood 1995; 86(suppl 1):182a.

Dr. Guillaume Dighiero, Unité d'Immuno-hématologie et d'Immunopathologie,
28, rue du Dr Roux, F–75015 Paris (France)
Tel. 33 1 45 68 82 10, Fax 33 1 45 68 89 51

Ferrarini M, Caligaris-Cappio F (eds): Human B Cell Populations.
Chem Immunol. Basel, Karger, 1997, vol 67, pp 102–113

....

B Cell Populations:
The Multiple Myeloma Model

Federico Caligaris-Cappio[a], *M. Grazia Gregoretti*[a], *Kenneth Nilsson*[b]

[a] Cattedra di Immunologia Clinica, Dipartimento di Scienze Biomediche e Oncologia
Umana, Università di Torino, Italy;
[b] Laboratory of Tumor Biology, Department of Pathology, University Hospital,
Uppsala, Sweden

B cell malignancies are regarded as clonal expansions of B lineage cells arrested at a particular stage of differentiation. Multiple myeloma (MM), which is characterized by the accumulation of plasmablasts-plasma cells that replace normal bone marrow (BM) and produce monoclonal immunoglobulins (Ig) and cytokines [1], has an ambiguous place in this conceptual framework because of several unusual features. First, normal plasma cells originate from different types of immune response, T-cell-dependent versus T-cell-independent and primary versus secondary, and accordingly, develop within different microenvironments in the presence of different specialized antigen (Ag)-presenting cells [2]. It may therefore be asked which plasma cell population is involved in the malignant process. Second, within a given MM clone various B cell phenotypes can be seen that favor the possibility of an ongoing intraclonal differentiation [3]. The question of which B cell differentiation window corresponds to the stage where the malignant cell is frozen leads, more specifically, to the controversial issue of whether a precursor plasma cell population exists and how it relates to the terminally differentiated plasma cell elements that form the bulk of malignant cells. Finally, the long-standing clinical considerations that MM is a BM disease which is widespread troughout the axial skeleton from the earliest recognizable stage, when very few plasma cells are seen in the peripheral blood (PB) [1], give rise to the question of whether the putative plasma cell precursors are circulating and which relationships they have with the BM microenvironment.

Numerous observations provided by both basic sciences and clinical investigation can help to place MM in a coherent perspective.

The Basics of Plasma Cell Development

Plasma cells originate from Ag-specific B cells after a number of developmental steps within different microenvironments. The process is controlled by the coordinated expression of gene programs for growth, differentiation, survival and death. These gene programs are regulated by a network of paracrine, autocrine and endocrine cytokines, acting in concert with signals elicited by cell-cell contacts and cell-extracellular matrix (ECM) interactions [2–6]. T-cell-independent responses take place in macrophage-rich areas, such as the red pulp of the spleen. T-cell-dependent primary responses develop in areas of extrafollicular secondary lymphoid tissues rich in T lymphocytes and interdigitating cells. T-cell-dependent secondary responses occur in germinal centers (GC) of secondary lymphoid follicles where follicular dendritic cells and T cells are present.

Virgin B cells undergo primary Ag stimulation in the extrafollicular areas of peripheral lymphoid organs, while memory B cells are recruited by secondary Ag response in lymphoid follicles where prominent GC progressively develop [7–9]. Within GC proliferating B cells (centroblasts) undergo the processes of somatic hypermutation leading to the generation of high affinity antibodies (Ab) and subsequently differentiate into noncycling centrocytes that switch their Ig isotype under the control of cytokines [8]. The unselected centrocytes die in situ by apoptosis and are disposed of by macrophages [8]. The selected centrocytes develop into either plasmablasts (plasma cell precursors) or into B memory cells that recirculate and may undergo another round of GC-based Ag-dependent activation, proliferation and differentiation [9]. GC-derived plasmablasts, that are characterized by a switched isotype and somatic hypermutations, have specific traffic commitments and migrate to the BM few days after the antigenic challenge to undergo terminal differentiation [8, 9]. The dogma that affinity maturation by somatic hypermutation occurs only within GC has recently been challenged by the results from studies of mice deficient in lymphotoxin-α. Such mice have neither lymph nodes, nor Peyer's patches and fail to form GC [10]. Still, when immunized with high doses of T-dependent Ag they produce a high affinity Ab response with somatic hypermutations like wild-type mice [10].

The Heterogeneity of Normal Plasma Cells and Its Relevance to Understanding the Origin of MM

The properties of plasma cells, including the morphology, Ig isotype, anatomical distribution and life span, vary according to the type of immune response that has led to their development [reviewed in 3]. Plasma cells generated in macrophage-rich areas after T-cell-independent Ag stimulation secrete IgM and are short-lived. A primary T-cell-dependent response in the extrafollicular areas also gives rise to short-lived plasma cells, which remain in the lymph node extramedullary regions. Secondary T-cell-dependent Ab responses lead to the production of IgG- or IgA-secreting plasma cells with a life span of few weeks. The dichotomy of B lineage cells into B1 or B2 B lymphocytes according to the presence (B1) or the absence (B2) of the surface CD5 molecule [11] has not yet provided phenotypic or molecular markers that properly discriminate B1-derived from B2-derived plasma cells.

Even if the steps of Ag processing and presentation occur only [or, at least, essentially, 10] in secondary lymphoid follicles [8], the BM is the major site where IgG and IgA are produced in T-cell-dependent secondary immune responses [4]. It is assumed that BM-seeking plasma cell precursors receive a differentiation signal at the time they come into contact with the BM stromal microenvironment [6, 9].

The properties of MM plasma cells and of the monoclonal Ig they produce may be used to understand to which plasma cell lineage MM should be affiliated. MM paraproteins may be directed against a wide variety of infectious agents, suggesting that the development of MM may be causally related to Ag stimulation [12–14]. Next, the Ig isotype of MM plasma cells is generally IgG or IgA, demonstrating that the predominant phenotype of MM tumor cells is that of a postswitch B cell [2]. Also, the clonal proliferation involves a cell population that has already passed through the stage of somatic hypermutation of Ig genes [15, 16]. As the process of Ig gene somatic mutation occurs in the GC of secondary follicles [8] following Ag stimulation and is coupled to the isotype switch, the above-mentioned observations indicate that peripheral lymphoid organ GC have a central role in the development of MM. By and large, the observation that MM is a neoplasm of plasmablasts-plasma cells that have a postswitch phenotype, show somatic mutations and may produce monoclonal Ig with targeted Ab activity might suggest that the evolution of MM is an Ag-triggered process. However, the specific causal Ag is generally unknown. An interesting difference has been observed between MM and monoclonal gammopathy of unknown significance (MGUS): ongoing somatic mutations are present in MGUS, but not in MM suggesting that MM is an Ag-selected while MGUS is an Ag-driven process [17].

Contrasting with the distribution of normal plasma cells, MM plasma cells localize uniquely within the BM [1–3]. Even if the lamina propria of the intestine contains more Ig-producing cells than all other tissues in the body, it is never a site where MM develops, not even the IgA-producing MM. Likewise, the involvement of the spleen and/or lymph nodes is typical of Waldenström's macroglobulinemia, but is very unusual in MM. The issue of whether MM plasma cell precursors are early BM stem cells or late peripheral B cells is misleading. The cell whose original transformation has ultimately generated the malignant plasma cell progeny observed in MM cannot be equated to the B cell population that disseminates the disease throughout the axial skeleton. The identity of the hypothetical MM stem cell is unknown. The information available on the B cell population that feeds the downstream compartment of plasma cells and disseminates the disease indicates that this population has been generated in peripheral lymphoid organs during secondary T-cell-dependent Ab response, is programmed to home to the BM and committed to differentiate in close association with the BM microenvironment [18]. The existing data suggest that the most likely candidate for the physiological B lymphocyte equivalent of the MM plasma cell precursor is either an activated B memory cell or a plasmablast [15–17, 19, 20].

The Phenotype of MM Plasma Cells

The precise phenotype of normal plasma cells is not fully established and, in general, their phenotypic features have been inferred from the phenotype of MM plasma cells [reviewed in 3]. The use of cytoplasmic expression of Ig with very little or no sIg as a reference marker has been used to scan the expression of surface molecules and has revealed two interesting phenotypic properties of plasma cells [21]. Conventional B cell surface markers are almost absent at the plasma cell level, as most B-specific and B-associated surface molecules are lost during the transition to the plasma cell stage, and a very large array of adhesion structures are acquired [3].

The best surface marker of plasma cells is CD38 whose expression is shared by both normal and MM plasma cells [22]. CD38 is not restricted to the B lineage nor is it stage-specific within the B cell lineage, as it is expressed both by plasma cells and by B blasts proliferating in the GC [3]. CD38 is related to the enzyme ADP-ribosyl cyclase that is involved in a pathway of intracellular Ca^{2+} mobilization that is distinct from the inositol 1,4,5-triphosphate one [23, 24]. CD38-mediated signal transduction may be crucial in the homeostatic control of lymphopoiesis [25] and agonistic monoclonal Ab to CD38 can be exploited for in vivo immunotherapy.

Normal plasma cells have been reported to be CD19-positive, while MM plasma cells are usually CD19-negative [22]. Immunophenotypic studies reveal that in a proportion of MM patients both BM plasma cells and some monoclonal B cells are CD10-positive [26, 27]. The PCR analysis with patient-specific Ig gene primers has shown that a small population of CD10-positive clonal cells exist in most patients with MM [28]. CD10 is expressed by early B lineage-committed cells in the BM [26], but also by GC B blasts and by activated B lymphocytes [27], again bringing the attention to the possible peripheral B cell nature of MM plasma cell precursors.

MM plasma cells express on the membrane adhesion molecules like H-CAM (CD44), ICAM-I (CD54), N-CAM (CD56), LFA-3 (CD58), the proteoglycan syndecan, a receptor for hyaluronan-mediated motility and frequently also CD11/CD18 [29–33]. It is conceivable that MM surface adhesion structures, by interacting with their homologous ligands in the BM microenvironment, may make it possible for malignant B cells to be entrapped within the BM stromal cell web, where they would be exposed to the locally produced cytokines [34–36]. Normal plasma cells are CD19-positive, CD56-negative, while MM plasma cells are almost invariably CD56-positive, thus suggesting a role for this molecule in the pathophysiology of the disease [34]. CD56 binds specifically to heparan sulfate, a member of the ECM protein family and it might thus be involved in the tumor cell-ECM protein interactions [37]. It has also been implicated in the homotypic adhesions of tumor cells which lead to the formation of MM plasma cell nodules and clusters [29, 34]. Consistent with this hypothesis, it has been reported that the loss of CD56 is associated with a more aggressive course of the disease and a tendency to disseminate plasma cells in PB [29].

Circulating Plasma Cells and Plasma Cell Precursors in MM

The observation that MM are widespread throughout the BM even when very few plasma cells are seen in the PB [1] has suggested that human MM, like murine plasmacytoma [38], may be disseminated by circulating clonogenic cells. Their existence is favored by different lines of evidence, including the presence of ciruclating B lymphocytes that express the MM paraprotein idiotype [39], the detection of a monoclonal Ig gene rearrangement with PB mononuclear cells [40], the identification of DNA-aneuploid cells in PB samples [1], the growth of plasma cell colonies from PB [41] and the induction of patients' mononuclear cells to plasma cell differentiation by cytokines [42]. However, the proportion of circulating clonal lymphocytes is debated [43], and the precise differentiation nature of putative plasma cell precursors has been challenged by other studies indicating that tumor-specific aneuploidy is not detected in CD19-positive B lymphoid cells [44].

The existence of circulating precursors is more a functional than a cytological concept, as their phenotype, notwithstanding several experimental approaches [see 45], is still ill-defined; the morphological (fig. 1) and functional flexibility of plasmablasts and plasma cells adds a further complication to the issue [46]. More specifically, it is yet unknown whether circulating plasma cell precursors in MM are plasmablasts or mature B cells. Likewise their precise traffic relationship with the plasma cell compartment is unknown. Two nonmutually exclusive possibilities exist: either that circulating precursor cells are 'coming' from the BM, spilling

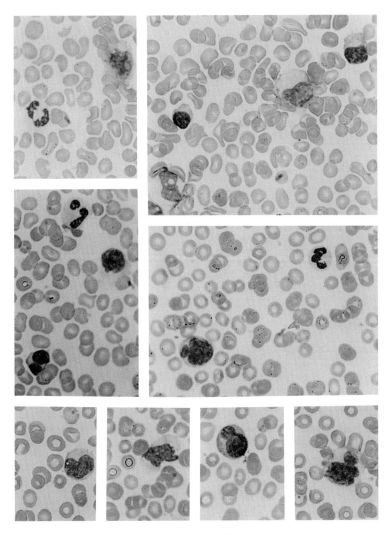

Fig. 1. The morphology of circulating CD38-positive, membrane light chain-restricted B cells in MM can be very variable.

over from an overcrowded environment, or that they are 'on their way' to the BM after having been primed in peripheral lymphoid organs. Recent data obtained in human MM by amplifying the complementary determining region (CDR) 3 have shown that the incidence of circulating monoclonal tumor-related cells is independent of both tumor burden and stage of disease [47] and may easily be detected even after successful autologous BM transplantation [48, 49]. By means of the CDR 3 amplification of rearranged heavy chain alleles the existence has been shown, within the BM of MM patients, of preswitch B cells clonally related to malignant plasma cells [19, 20]. This population is extremely small, shows somatic hypermutations and is not seen in PB where only postswitch B cells, with the tumor VDJ sequences bound to $C\alpha$ or $C\gamma$, have been detected [19]. The precise place of BM preswitch cells in the evolution of MM clone is unknown. Interestingly, a similar event has been shown to occur in the rare cases of IgG-positive B-chronic lymphocytic leukemia, where mRNA transcripts coding for patient-specific heavy chain variable region have been found to be linked to $C\mu$ and $C\alpha$ heavy chain genes [50]. Collectively, these data suggest that BM preswitch cells might represent clonal B memory cells which have not yet completed their full differentiation and are still waiting for the switch process to occur. Alternatively, they can be regarded as a 'blind alley' in the natural history of the malignant clone. An entirely speculative view is that if somatic hypermutations and differentiation may occur in the absence of GC [10], the BM may be the place where the whole life of MM clones not only has an end but also its beginning.

BM Microenvironment and MM

BM microenvironment regulates B lymphopoiesis [51, 52]. Microenvironmental stromal cells play an essential role in the growth of plasma cell tumors both in mice [53] and in humans [54]. MM BM stromal cells are well equipped with a large series of adhesion and ECM proteins that mediate homotypic and heterotypic interactions and provide anchorage sites to cells selectively exposed to locally released growth factors [18]. MM BM stromal cells also produce cytokines, like IL-6, known to play a crucial role in the evolution of the disease [55]. The physical contact between MM plasma cells and BM stromal cells increases IL-6 production [56]: one of the key regulatory elements for MM plasma cell-induced IL-6 transcription in BM stromal cells is activation of NF-kB [57]. In vitro, the growth of human MM cell lines can be improved by IL-6 or is dependent on IL-6-producing feeder cells [58–60]. IL-6 is a potent growth factor for murine hybridomas and plasmacytomas and, at present, is the most relevant growth factor known not only for human MM cell lines, but also for fresh MM samples [57–61]. Consistent with these in vitro findings, high levels of IL-6 are observed in the sera of patients with aggressive or progressive MM [62, 63], and the infusion of anti-IL-6 Ab in patients with plasma cell leukemia or MM refractory to therapy has decreased the size of the plasma cell pool and prevented the proliferative activity of plasma cells [64]. IL-6, besides promoting B cell proliferation and differentiation, has an important osteoclast-activating factor role [65]. Other cytokines, like granulocyte-macrophage colony-stimulating factor, IL-1, IL-3 and IL-5, frequently in synergy with IL-6, may increase the ^{3}H-Tdr incorporation of purified MM plasma cells cultured in vitro [60, 66, 67] and, recently, IGF-1 has been shown to be a growth and survival factor for myeloma cell lines [68].

MM malignant plasma cells produce a number of cytokines that include IL-1β, tumor necrosis factor-β, monocyte-macrophage colony-stimulating factor, that activate stromal, accessory cells and osteoblasts and also have a significant osteoclast-activating factor activity [69–72]. Activated T cells, fibroblasts and accessory cells are able to produce several cytokines potentially relevant to the growth of MM [reviewed in 18].

These experimental findings, linked to clinical observations, have led to the attractive hypothesis that a self-maintaining series of mutually interacting paracrine loops occurs between the malignant B cell clone and the BM microenvironment that lead to the production of ever-increasing amounts of cytokines and may explain the progression of MM [18].

gp 130-Linked Cytokines and MM: The Lesson from MM Cell Lines

A minority of human MM cell lines autonomously produce small amounts of IL-6, while it is debated whether and to what extent fresh MM plasma cells may also produce IL-6 [58, 73]. In any case, malignant MM plasma cells express IL-6 receptor (IL-6R) [59, 60]. The IL-6R is a complex where the binding of IL-6 to IL-6R triggers the association of a nonligand binding 130-kD signal-transducing molecule [61, 74], gp130, a transducer common to several distantly related cytokines [74]. This family of cytokines includes IL-6, oncostatin M (OM), leukemia-inhibiting factor, ciliary neurotrophic factor, IL-11 and cardiotrophin-1 [74]. Besides IL-6, a number of cytokines that use gp130 as common signal transducer pathway, such as ciliary neurothrophic factor, leukemia-inhibiting factor and OM, are potent in vitro growth factors for MM [61, 74]; the OM-induced signaling involves the Janus kinase JAK2 [75].

The ability of IL-6 to induce osteoclast differentiation is also based upon signal transduction mediated by IL-6R which is expressed on osteoblastic cells but not on osteoclast precursors [65]. The nature of these precursors and their relationships with the BM microenvironment in MM still have to be fully elucidated. The precise molecular definition of the interactions between the different cell populations that are involved in the evolution of MM will allow a more proper definition of the events that might hopefully be influenced for therapeutic purposes.

Acknowledgement

This work was supported by AIRC, Milano and by PF ACRO, CNR, Roma and by the Swedish Cancer Society. MGG is the recipient of an AIRC fellowship. The secretarial assistance of Mrs. G. Tessa, Fondazione R. Favretto, is gratefully acknowledged.

References

1   Barlogie B, Epstein J, Selvanayagam P, Alexanian R: Plasma cell myeloma: New biological insights and advances in therapy: Blood 1989;73:865–879.
2   MacLennan ICM, Chan EYT: The origin of bone marrow plasma cells; in Obrams GI, Potter M (eds): Epidemiology and Biology of Multiple Myeloma, Berlin, Springer, 1991, pp 129–135.
3   Caligaris-Cappio F, Gregoretti MG: Basic concepts: Plasma cells in multiple myeloma; in Durie BGM, Gahrton G (eds): Multiple Myeloma. London, Arnold, 1996, pp 22–35.
4   Benner R, Hijmans W, Haajman JJ: The bone marrow: The major source of serum immunoglobulins, but still a neglected site of antibody formation. Clin Exp Immunol 1981;46:1–8.
5   Ho F, Lortan J, Khan M, MacLennan ICM: Distinct short-lived and long-lived antibody-producing cell populations. Eur J Immunol 1986;16:1297–1301.
6   DiLosa RM, Maeda K, Masuda A, Szakal AK, Tew JG: Germinal center B cells and antibody production in the bone marrow. J Immunol 1991;146:4071–4077.
7   MacLennan ICM, Gray D: Antigen-driven selection of virgin and memory B cells. Immunol Rev 1986;91:61–85.
8   Kelsoe G: Life and death in germinal centers (Redux). Immunity 1996;4:107–111.
9   Liu YJ, Johnson GD, Gordon J, MacLennan ICM: Germinal centres in T-cell dependent antibody responses. Immunol Today 1992;13:17–21.
10   Matsumoto M, Lo SF, Carruthers CJL, Min J, Mariathasan S, Huang G, Plas DR, Martin SM, Geha RS, Nahm MH, Chaplin DD: Affinity maturation without germinal centres in lymphotoxin-α deficient mice. Nature 1996;382:462–466.
11   Kantor AB: The development and repertoire of B-1 cells (CD5 B cells). Immunol Today 1991;12: 389–391.
12   Potter M: Myeloma proteins (M-components) with antibody-like activity. N Engl J Med 1971;284: 831–838.
13   Seligmann M, Brouet JC: Antibody activity of human myeloma globulins. Semin Hematol 1973;10: 163–177.
14   Konrad RJ, Kricka LJ, Goodman DBP, Goldman J, Silberstein LE: Myeloma-associated paraprotein directed against the HIV-1 p24 antigen in an HIV-1-seropositive patient. N Engl J Med 1993; 328:1817–1819.
15   Bakus MHC, Heirman C, Van Riet I, Van Camp B, Thielemans K: Evidence that multiple myeloma Ig heavy chain VDJ genes contain somatic mutations but show no intraclonal variation. Blood 1992;80:2326–2335.
16   Vescio RA, Cao J, Hong CH, Lee JC, Wu CH, Der-Danielian M, Wu V, Newman R, Lichtenstein AK, Berenson JR: Myeloma Ig heavy chain V region sequences reveal prior antigenic selection and marked somatic mutation but not intraclonal diversity. J Immunol 1995;155:2487–2497.
17   Sahota SS, Leo R, Hamblin TJ, Stevenson FK: Ig VH gene mutational patterns indicate different tumor cell status in human myeloma and monoclonal gammopathy of undetermined significance. Blood 1996;87:746–755.
18   Caligaris-Cappio F, Gregoretti MG, Ghia P, Bergui L: In vitro growth of human multiple myeloma: Implications for biology and therapy. Hematol Oncol Clin North Am 1992;6:257–271.
19   Billadeau D, Ahmann G, Greipp P, Van Ness B: The bone marrow of multiple myeloma patients contains B cell populations at different stages of differentiation that are clonally related to the malignant plasma cell. J Exp Med 1993;178:1023–1031.

20   Corradini P, Boccadoro M, Voena C, Pileri A: Evidence for a bone marrow B cell transcribing malignant plasma cell VDJ joined to Cμ sequence in IgG and IgA secreting multiple myelomas. J Exp Med 1993;178:1091–1096.

21   Anderson KC, Park EK, Bates MP, Leonard CF, Hardy R, Schlossman SF, Nadler LM: Antigens on human plasma cells identified by monoclonal antibodies. J Immunol 1992;130:1132–1138.

22   Harada H, Kawano MM, Huang N, Harada Y, Iwato K, Tanabe O, Tanaka H, Sakai A, Asaoku H, Kuramoto A: Phenotypic difference of normal plasma cells from mature myeloma cells. Blood 1993;81:2658–2663.

23   States DJ, Walseth TF, Lee HC: Similarities in amino acid sequences of aplysia ADP-ribosyl cyclase and human lymphocyte antigen CD38. Trends Biochem Sci 1992;17:495–499.

24   Galione A: Cyclic ADP-ribose: A new way to control calcium. Science 1993;259:325–326.

25   Kitanaka A, Ito C, Nishigaki H, Campana D: CD38-mediated growth suppression of B-cell progenitors requires activation of phosphatidylinositol 3-kinase and involves its association with the protein product of the c-C=cbl protooncogene. Blood 1996;88:590–598.

26   Caligaris-Cappio F, Bergui L, Tesio L, Pizzolo G, Malavasi F, Chilosi M, Campana D, van Camp B, Janossy G: Identification of malignant plasma cell precursors in the bone marrow of multiple myeloma. J Clin Invest 1985;76:1243–1251.

27   Warburton P, Joshua DE, Gibson J, Brown RD: CD10-(CALLA)-positive lymphocytes in myeloma: Evidence that they are a malignant precursor population and are of germinal centre origin. Leuk Lymphoma 1989;1:11–20.

28   Cao J, Vescio RA, Rettig MB, Hong CH, Kim A, Lichtenstein AK, Berenson JR: A CD10-positive subset of malignant cells is identified in multiple myeloma using PCR with patient-specific immunoglobulin gene primers. Leukemia 1995;9:1948–1953.

29   Van Camp B, Durie BGM, Spier C, DeWaele M, Van Riet I, Vela E, Frutiger Y, Richter L, Grogan TM: Plasma cells in multiple myeloma express a natural killer cell-associated antigen: CD56 (NKH-1; Leu-19). Blood 1990;76:377–382.

30   Lewinsohn DM, Nagler A, Ginzton N, Greenberg P, Butcher EC: Hematopoietic progenitor cells expression of the H-CAM (CD44) homing-associated adhesion molecule. Blood 1990;76:589–594.

31   Uchiyama H, Barut BA, Chauhan D, Cannistra SA, Anderson KC: Characterization of adhesion molecules on human myeloma cell lines. Blood 1992;80:2306–2314.

32   Turley EA, Belch AJ, Poppema S, Pilarski L: Expression and function of a receptor for hyaluronan-mediated motility on normal and malignant B lymphocytes. Blood 1993;81:446–453.

33   Ridley RC, Xiao H, Hata H, Woodliff J, Epstein J, Sanderson RD: Expression of syndecan regulates human myeloma plasma cell adhesion to type I collagen. Blood 1993;81:767–774.

34   Van Riet I, Van Camp B: The involvement of adhesion molecules in the biology of multiple myeloma. Leuk Lymphoma 1993;9:441–452.

35   Thiery JP, Boyer B: The junction between cytokines and cell adhesion. Curr Opin Cell Biol 1992;4:782–792.

36   Hynes RO: Integrins: Versatility, modulation and signalling in cell adhesion. Cell 1992;69:11–25.

37   Juliano RL, Haskill S: Signal transduction from the extracellular matrix. J Cell Biol 1993;120:577–585.

38   Lynch RG, Rohrer JM, Odermatt B, Gebel M, Autry JR, Hoover RG: Immunoregulation of murine myeloma cell growth and differentiation: A monoclonal model of B cell differentiation. Immunol Rev 1977;48:45–73.

39   Osterborg A, Steinitz M, Lewin N, Bergenbrant S, Holm G, Lefvert AK, Mellstedt H: Establishment of idiotype bearing B-lymphocyte clones from a patient with monoclonal gammopathy. Blood 1991;78:2642–2649.

40   Berenson J, Wong R, Kim K, Brown N, Lichtenstein A: Evidence of peripheral blood B lymphocyte but not T lymphocyte involvement in multiple myeloma. Blood 1987;70:1550–1553.

41   Hamburger AW, Salmon SE: Primary bioassay of human myeloma stem cells. J Clin Invest 1977;60:846–854.

42   Bergui L, Schena M, Gaidano R, Riva M, Caligaris-Cappio F: Interleukin 3 and interleukin 6 synergistically promote the proliferation and differentiation of malignant plasma cell precursors in multiple myeloma. J Exp Med 1989;170:613–618.

43   Chen BJ, Epstein J: Circulating clonal lymphocytes in myeloma constitute a minor subpopulation of B cells. Blood 1996;87:1972–1976.
44   McSweeney PA, Wells DA, Shults KE, Nash RA, Bensinger WI, Buckner CD, Loken MR: Tumor-specific aneuploidy not detected in CD19+ B-lymphoid cells from myeloma patients in a multidimensional flow cytometric analysis. Blood 1996;88:622–632.
45   Jensen GS, Belch AR, Mant MJ, Ruether BA, Pilarski LM: Expression of multiple adhesion molecules on circulating monoclonal B cells in myeloma. Curr Top Microbiol Immunol 1992;182:187–193.
46   Nilsson K, Pontén J: Classification and biological nature of established human hematopoietic cell lines. Int J Cancer 1975;15:321–341.
47   Billadeau D, Quam L, Thomas W, Kay N, Greipp P, Kyle R, Oken MM, Van Ness B: Detection and quantitation of malignant cells in the peripheral blood of multiple myeloma patients. Blood 1992; 80:1818–1824.
48   Corradini P, Voena C, Astolfi M, Ladetto M, Tarella C, Boccadoro M, Pileri A: High-dose sequential chemoradiotherapy in multiple myeloma: Residual tumor cells are detectable in bone marrow and peripheral blood harvests and after autografting. Blood 1995;85:1596–1602.
49   Lemoli R, Fortuna A, Motta MR, Rizzi S, Giudice V, Nannetti A, Martinelli G, Cavo M, Amabile M, Mangianti S, Fogli M, Conte R, Tura S: Concomitant mobilization of plasma cells and hematopoietic progenitors into peripheral blood of multiple myeloma patients: Positive selection and transplantation of enriched CD34+ cells to remove circulating tumor cells. Blood 1996;87:1625–1634.
50   Dono M, Hashimoto S, Fais F, Trejo V, Allen SL, Lichtman SM, Schulman P, Vinciguerra VP, Sellars B, Gregersen PK, Ferrarini M, Chiorazzi N: Evidence for progenitors of chronic lymphocytic leukemia B cells that undergo intraclonal differentiation and differentiation. Blood 1996;87: 1586–1594.
51   Kinkade P, Lee G, Pietrangeli CE, Hayashi SH, Gimble J: Cells and molecules that regulate B lymphopoiesis in bone marrow. Annu Rev Immunol 1989;7:111–143.
52   Rolink A, Melchers F: Generation and regeneration of cells of the B-lymphocyte lineage. Curr Opin Immunol 1993;5:207–217.
53   Degrassi A, Hilbert DM, Rudikoff S, Anderson AO, Potter M, Coon HG: In vitro culture of primary plasmacytomas requires stromal cell feeder layers. Proc Natl Acad Sci USA 1993;90:2060–2064.
54   Caligaris-Cappio F, Bergui L, Gregoretti MG, Gaidano G, Gaboli M, Schena M, Zambonin-Zallone A, Marchisio PC: Role of bone marrow stromal cells in the growth of human multiple myeloma. Blood 1991;77:2688–2693.
55   Klein B, Zhang XG, Jourdan M, Content J, Houssiau F, Aarden L, Piechaczyk M, Bataille R: Paracrine rather than autocrine regulation of myeloma-cell growth and differentiation by interleukin-6. Blood 1989;73:517–526.
56   Lokhorst HM, Lamme T, deSmet M, Klein S, de Weger RA, van Oers R, Bloem AC: Primary tumor cells of myeloma patients induce interleukin-6 secretion in long-term bone marrow cultures. Blood 1994;84:2269–2274.
57   Chauhan D, Uchiyama H, Akbarali Y, Urashima M, Yamamoto KI, Libermann TA, Anderson KC: Multiple myeloma cell adhesion-induced interleukin-6 expression in bone marrow stromal cells involves activation of NF-kB. Blood 1996;87:1104–1112.
58   Jernberg H, Pettersson M, Kishimoto T, Nilsson K: Heterogeneity in response to interleukin 6 (IL-6), expression of IL-6 and IL-6 receptor mRNA in a panel of established human multiple myeloma cell lines. Leukemia 1991;5:255–265.
59   Nilsson K, Jernberg H, Pettersson M: IL-6 as a growth factor for human multiple myeloma cells – A short overview. Curr Top Microbiol Immunol 1990;166:3–8.
60   Nilsson K: The control of growth in human multiple myeloma cell-lines; in Dammacco F, Barlogie B (eds): Multiple Myeloma and Related Disorders. Ares-Serono Symposia, Geneva, 1994, vol 4, pp 83–89.
61   Klein B, Zhang XG, Lu ZY, Bataille R: Interleukin-6 in human multiple myeloma. Blood 1995;85: 863–872.

62   Bataille R, Jourdan M, Zhang XG, Klein B: Serum levels of interleukin-6, a potent myeloma cell growth factor, as a reflection of disease severity in plasma cell dyscrasias. J Clin Invest 1989;84: 2008–2011.

63   Merico F, Bergui L, Gregoretti MG, Ghia P, Aimo G, Lindley IJD, Caligaris-Cappio F: Cytokines involved in the progression of multiple myeloma. Clin Exp Immunol 1993;92:27–31.

64   Klein B, Wijdenes J, Zhang XG, Jourdan M, Boiron JM, Brochier J, Liautard J, Merlin M, Clement C, Morel-Fournier B, Lu ZY, Mannoni P, Sany J, Bataille R: Murine anti-interleukin-6 monoclonal antibody therapy for a patient with plasma cell leukemia. Blood 1991;78:1198–1204.

65   Udagawa N, Takahashi N, Katagiri T, Tamura T, Wada S, Findlay DM, Martin TJ, Hirota H, Taga T, Kishimoto T, Suda T: Interleukin (IL)-6 induction of osteoclast differentiation depends on IL-6 receptors expressed on osteoblastic cells but not on osteoclast progenitors. J Exp Med 1995;182: 1461–1468.

66   Anderson KC, Jones RM, Morimoto C, Leavitt P, Barut A: Response patterns of purified myeloma cells to hematopoietic growth factors. Blood 1989;73:1915–1924.

67   Zhang XCG, Bataille R, Jourdan M, Saeland S, Banchereau J, Mannoni P, Klein B: GM-CSF synergizes with interleukin-6 in supporting the proliferation of human myeloma cells. Blood 1990; 76:2599–2605.

68   Georgii-Hemming P, Jernberg-Wiklund H, Ljunggren Ö, Nilsson K: IGF-I is a growth and survival factor in human myeloma cell lines. Blood, in press.

69   Cozzolino F, Torcia M, Aldinucci D, Rubartelli A, Miliani A, Shaw AR, Lansdorp PM, Di Gugliel-mo R: Production of interleukin-1 by bone marrow myeloma cells. Blood 1989;74:380–387.

70   Mundy GR, Raisz LG, Cooper RA, Schechter GP, Salmon SE: Evidence for the secretion of an osteoclast stimulating factor in myeloma. N Engl J Med 1974;291:1041–1046.

71   Ross Garrett I, Durie BGM, Nedwin GE, Gillespie A, Bringman T, Sabatini M, Bertolini DR, Mundy GR: Production of lymphotoxin, a bone-resorbing cytokine, by cultured human myeloma cells. N Engl J Med 1987;317:526–532.

72   Nakamura M, Merchav S, Carter A, Ernst TJ, Demetri GD, Furukawa Y, Anderson K, Freedman AS, Griffin JD: Expression of a novel 3.5-kb macrophage colony-stimulating factor transcript in human myeloma cells. J Immunol 1989;143:3543–3547.

73   Kawano M, Hirano T, Matsuda T, Taga T, Horii Y, Iwato K, Asaoku H, Tang B, Tanabe O, Tanaka H, Kuramoto A, Kishimoto T: Autocrine generation and requirement of BSF-2/IL-6 for human multiple myeloma. Nature 1988;332:83–86.

74   Kishimoto T, Akira S, Narazaki M, Taga T: Interleukin-6 family of cytokines and gp130. Blood 1995;86:1243–1254.

75   Chauhan D, Kharbanda SM, Ogata A, Urashima M, Frank D, Malik N, Kufe DW, Anderson KC: Oncostatin M induces association of Grb2 with Janus kinase JAK2 in multiple myeloma cells. J Exp Med 1995;182:1801–1806.

F. Caligaris-Cappio, MD, Cattedra di Immunologia Clinica, Via Genova 3, I–10126 Torino (Italy)
Tel. +39 11 6637230, Fax +39 11 6637238, E-Mail Caligari@golgi.molinette.unito.it

Ferrarini M, Caligaris-Cappio F (eds): Human B Cell Populations.
Chem Immunol. Basel, Karger, 1997, vol 67, pp 114–132

....

Regulation of Human B Cell Growth and Differentiation: Lessons from the Primary Immunodeficiencies

Robin E. Callard, Susan H. Smith, David J. Matthews

Immunobiology Unit, Institute of Child Health, London, UK

Introduction

Genetic defects have been identified in a number of primary immunodeficiencies with either autosomal or X-linked patterns of inheritance. These include mutations in genes coding for intracellular signalling proteins, adhesion molecules, cell surface interaction antigens, cytokine receptors and various enzymes (table 1).

Each of these immunodeficiencies can be considered as a naturally occurring gene inactivation model with a well-characterised disease phenotype. The molecular characterisation of the proteins coded for by the defective genes has led to important advances in our understanding of both the immunodeficiency itself and the basic cellular and molecular mechanisms that determine normal immune function. Ultimately, these studies of basic immune mechanisms in immunodeficiency and their clinical sequelae will lead to new forms of treatment including gene replacement therapy.

X-Linked Immunodeficiencies

In the past 5 years the genes responsible for six of the eight known X-linked immunodeficiencies have been identified (table 2). These are X-linked severe combined immunodeficiency (SCIDX1), X-linked agammaglobulinaemia (XLA), X-linked hyper-IgM syndrome (HIGM1), Wiskott-Aldrich syndrome (WAS), X-linked chronic granulomatous disease (CGD), and properdin deficien-

Table 1. Gene defects in primary immunodeficiencies

Disease	Phenotype	Defective protein
Lymphocyte activation and maturation		
Autosomal recessive SCID	Low/absent T and B cells	RAG1, RAG2
Jak3 SCID	Low/absent T and NK cells	Jak3
XSCID	Low/absent T and NK cells	γc-chain
XLA	Low/absent B cells	Btk
CD3γ, CD3ε deficiency	Defective T activation	CD3γ, CD3ε
ZAP70 deficiency	Defective T activation	ZAP70
HIGM1	Absent Th activity	CD40L
Antigen Presentation		
HLA class I gene	Low CD8+ and NK	TAP2
HLA class II gene	Low CD4+	CIITA, RFX5
Control of cell death		
fas deficiency	Lymphoproliferation and autoimmunity	Fas
Toxicity		
ADA deficiency	T and B lymphopenia	ADA
PNP deficiency	T cell lymphopenia	PNP
Phagocytic deficiencies		
LAD (CD18)	Defective leucocyte adhesion	β-Integrin
CGD	Defective intracellular killing	gp91^{phox}, p22^{phox}, p47^{phox}, p67^{phox}
Others		
WAS	Lymphocyte and platelet defects	WASP
AT	DNA repair defect	ATM

ADA = Adenosine deaminase; PNP = purine nucleoside phosphorylase; LAD = leukocyte adhesion defect; CGD = X-linked chronic granulomatous disease; WAS = Wiskott-Aldrich syndrome; AT = ataxia telangectasia.

cy. The genes responsible for X-linked lymphoproliferative disease (Duncan's syndrome) and XLA with growth hormone deficiency have yet to be identified.

In this chapter, two examples of X-linked immunodeficiencies (SCIDX1 and HIGM1) are discussed to show how these lessons from nature have enhanced our understanding of the molecular mechanisms that regulate the immune system.

Table 2. X-linked immunodeficiencies

Immunodeficiency	Gene	Function
HIGM1	CD40L	T cell surface interaction
XLA	Btk	Cytoplasmic PTK
SCIDX1	γc-chain	Cytokine receptor
Wiskott-Aldrich syndrome	was	Signalling protein
Chronic granulomatous disease	gp91-phox	NADPH oxidase
Properdin deficiency	Properdin	Alternative complement
X-linked lymphoproliferative syndrome	?	?
XLA with growth hormone deficiency	?	?

PTK = Protein tyrosine kinase.

SCIDX1 and the IL-2 Receptor γ-Chain

The molecular characterisation of SCIDX1 has had a major impact on basic immunology. This is a devastating immunodeficiency characterised by profoundly defective cellular and humoral immunity resulting in greatly increased susceptibility to infection and is uniformly fatal by 1–2 years of age unless treated by bone marrow transplantation [1, 2]. Affected boys have markedly reduced or absent T cells, but B cells are often present in normal or even increased numbers [2]. B cells from SCIDX1 patients can secrete immunoglobulin on stimulation with pokeweed mitogen in the presence of normal T cells, but other in vitro assays have uncovered defective responses to mitogens and cytokines [2]. In obligate carriers of SCIDX1, the X chromosome is non-randomly inactivated in T cells, and may be non-randomly inactivated in B cells, neutrophils and monocytes consistent with a gene expressed in most if not all haematopoietic cell lineages [3, 4]. The gene responsible for SCIDX1 has been mapped to Xq13 [5–7]. The gene coding for the IL-2 receptor γ-chain (IL-2Rγ), now called the common γ-chain (γc-chain) also maps to this locus [8, 9] and mutations in the γc-chain gene are responsible for SCIDX1 [8, 10].

The γc-Chain and the IL-2 Receptor
The IL-2 receptor (IL-2R) is a complex of three distinct polypeptide subunits [11]. The α-chain (Tac, p55 or CD25) binds IL-2 with low affinity (K_d 10^{-8} M) and a short dissociation half-life of 1.7 s [12]. The larger β-chain (p75, CD122) also binds IL-2 with low affinity (K_d 10^{-7} M), whereas the γ-chain (γc-chain, p64) does not bind IL-2. The heterotrimeric complex of the α/β/γ-chains binds IL-2

with high affinity (K_d $10^{-11} M$). Receptor complexes of the α/β-chain also bind IL-2 with high affinity (K_d $10^{-10} M$) but may not deliver a mitogenic signal, whereas complexes of the β/γ-chain bind IL-2 (K_d $10^{-9} M$) and can deliver a mitogenic signal [12]. The α-chain has two extracellular domains with homology to the complement control protein also known as the 'sushi domain' or GP-I motif. It has a very short intracellular region and does not signal. The IL-15Rα chain has homology with the IL-2Rα chain (CD25) and together they define a new cytokine receptor family [13]. The IL-2Rβ and γc-chains are both members of the cytokine receptor superfamily.

Neither the IL-2Rβ nor γ-chains have intrinsic kinase activity and the phosphorylation events triggered by IL-2 binding and receptor heterodimerisation depend on activation of cellular protein kinases [14–17] which phosphorylate cellular proteins including the IL-2Rβ and γc-chains themselves [18, 19] and activation of c-fos, c-jun, c-myb and c-myc [20–23] culminating in lymphocyte proliferation and differentiation. Heterodimerisation of the IL-2Rβ and γc-chains is also thought to bring Jak1 and Jak3 kinases into close proximity allowing cross-phosphorylation and activation of their catalytic domains followed by phosphorylation of STAT3 and STAT5 [24, 25]. The importance of the γc-chain in signal transduction by IL-2 has been established in fibroblast transfection experiments showing that its presence in the IL-2R complex is required for protein tyrosine phosphorylation and induction of c-myc, c-fos and c-jun [26], and activation of Jak3 [27]. Receptor internalisation following IL-2 binding also requires a functional γc-chain [28]. Truncations of the γc-chain gene and point mutations causing loss of Jak3 association with the γc-chain have been found in SCIDX1 [29]. Interestingly, mutations in the Jak3 gene have been found in an autosomal form of SCID consistent with the importance of this signalling pathway for responses to IL-2 [30].

Other Cytokine Receptors That Use the γc-Chain

The γc-chain is also known to be a functional component of the receptors for IL-4 [31, 32], IL-7 [33], IL-9 [34] and IL-15 [35]. It is required for tyrosine phosphorylation of the insulin receptor substrate-1 (IRS-1) and IRS-2 (4PS) in response to IL-4 [32], and efficient internalisation of the IL-7R on binding of IL-7 [36]. In transfection experiments, proliferation of mouse F7 cells to IL-4 or IL-7 required expression of the γc-chain in addition to the IL-4R or IL-7R [37]. An antibody to the murine γc-chain blocks binding and inhibits IL-9 responses by IL-9-dependent cell lines [34]. These experiments clearly show that the γc-chain is a signalling component of the receptors for IL-2, IL-4, IL-7 and IL-9.

The fact that the γc-chain is a functional component of the receptors for IL-2, IL-4, IL-7, IL-9 and IL-15 suggests that signalling elements dependent on the γc-chain may be common to all of them. IL-2, IL-4, IL-7, IL-9 and IL-15 all activate

Jak1 and Jak3 [24, 38]. However, whereas IL-2, IL-15 and IL-7 activate STAT3 and STAT5 [24, 25, 39], IL-4 and IL-13 activate STAT6 and not STAT5 [24, 40]. The activation of the same STATs by IL-2, IL-7 and IL-15 can be explained by the presence of similar tyrosine-phosphorylated motifs that serve as STAT5 docking sites in the cytoplasmic domain of the β-chain of the IL-7R and the common β-chain of the IL-2R and IL-15R [35, 39]. STAT6 on the other hand binds to a docking site on the IL-4Rα chain which is also a component of the IL-13R [41]. Significantly, although IL-13 activates STAT6, it does not activate Jak3 [42] suggesting that the specificity of STAT6 activation is due to its docking site on the IL-4Rα chain and not the activation of Jak3. It will be interesting to determine whether the recently identified IL-13 binding protein(s) [43–46] which associate with the IL-4Rα chain to form the IL-13R complex are themselves able to bind and activate an as yet unidentified Jak protein, or some other kinase which can activate STAT6.

γc-Chain Mutations in SCIDX1

More than 30 different γc-chain gene mutations in unrelated SCIDX1 patients have been described. These include point mutations giving rise to single amino acid substitutions, deletions which may cause frame shifts with premature stop codons giving rise to a predicted truncated protein, and splice site mutations. In a recent study of γc-chain gene mutations in 6 X-SCID patients by DiSanto et al. [47], loss of most or all high-affinity IL-2 binding sites in 4 of them was due to point mutations in the extracellular domain resulting in loss of tertiary structure or ligand binding. Another mutation consisting of a 4-bp deletion in the transmembrane domain of the γc-chain also resulted in loss of cytokine binding which may be explained by a loss of structural integrity affecting membrane anchoring. Loss of binding in the sixth example was due to absence of γc-chain mRNA and protein expression [47]. In a similar study, Ishii et al. [48] described three γc-chain mutations in SCIDX1. One of these was an A->V_{156} substitution in the loop joining the CK and FIII domains just distal to the leucine zipper motif and resulted in loss of high-affinity IL-2 binding sites. This residue is close to the site which binds the D helix of IL-2 [49] and the A->V mutation may disrupt cytokine binding, although a loss of structural integrity may also prevent association with the other receptor subunit components. A second mutation consisting of a 2-bp deletion causing a frame shift of the coding region in the SH2 domain of the cytoplasmic domain resulted in a loss of ability to signal but did not affect cytokine binding. The third mutation was a deletion of exon 2 with a frame shift and no detectable γc-chain expression. An E->K_{68} mutation described by Markiewicz also results in loss of high affinity binding sites without loss of γc-chain mRNA. Although γc-chain protein expression may occur in this patient, no γc-chain expression could be detected by antibody staining in one of our patients with the same mutation.

Three other nonsense mutations resulted in reduced mRNA expression with abnormal splicing in one with no functional protein.

Some γc-chain gene mutations may result in only partial loss of γc-chain function giving rise to a less severe or variable disease phenotype [50]. In one large family, affected boys had chronic bacterial and viral infections but were not affected with *Pneumocystis carinii* typical of SCIDX1, and some lived into late childhood or early adulthood [51]. Serum Ig levels were normal. CD4+ and CD8+ numbers were decreased but not as low as usually seen in SCIDX1. A point mutation giving rise to a Leu_{293}->Gln substitution in the cytoplasmic domain of the γc-chain was found in this family [52]. The effect of this mutation on γc-chain association with other components of the receptor complex or the effects on signalling have not yet been determined. It will be interesting to see whether the mutation results in partial receptor dysfunction for IL-2, IL-4, IL-7, IL-9 and IL-15, or loss of activity in only some of these receptors. The latter is a possibility as it is known that the epitope on the γc-chain defined by monoclonal antibodies required for binding IL-2 and IL-7 is distinct from the epitope required for binding of IL-4 [53].

Another family with a mild form of SCIDX1 has been described by DiSanto et al. [54]. Affected boys in this family suffered from recurrent infection, severe diarrhoea and failure to thrive [55]. Serum Ig levels and peripheral T cell, B cell and NK cell numbers were normal, but specific antibody responses were defective [47, 54]. T cell receptor β-chain expression was oligoclonal suggesting that the defect allowed the generation of a limited number of peripheral T cell clones [54]. Analysis of γc-chain cDNA and genomic sequences revealed a splice site mutation which gave rise to two γc-chain transcripts [54]. One of these was an abundant non-functional form with an insertion of a small intronic sequence. The other much less abundant form was functional and produced a γc-chain with a single D_{39}->N amino acid substitution. High-affinity IL-2R expression was 5-fold lower than in normal controls consistent with the abundancy of the non-functional transcript. Loss of function may be due to loss of high-affinity receptors and/or the point mutation in the γc-chain expressed in the residual high affinity receptors.

These examples will no doubt encourage other investigators to consider γc-chain mutations in atypical combined immunodeficiencies with an X-linked pedigree. Characterisation of γc-chain gene mutations that give rise to milder forms of SCIDX1 will prove invaluable for determining the functional sites on the γc-chain and the role of these sites in cytokine binding and signalling.

The Effect of γc-Chain Gene Mutations on SCIDX1 Lymphocyte Function

Cell-mediated and humoral immunity are typically defective in SCIDX1, and T cell numbers are very low or absent, although B cell numbers are usually normal. In contrast, autosomal SCID patients unable to make IL-2 [56], and mice in which the IL-2 gene [57], IL-4 gene [58], or both IL-2 and IL-4 genes [59] have been inactivated by targeted gene disruption have normal numbers of T cells and do not show the same immunological abnormalities as SCIDX1. The profound cell-mediated and humoral immunodeficiency in SCIDX1 is therefore thought to be due to the combined inability to respond to IL-2, IL-4, IL-7, IL-9 and IL-15. This conclusion itself raises some problematical questions. For example, IL-7 and IL-9 are involved in neuronal differentiation in the hippocampus yet abnormal brain development or function does not appear to be a feature of SCIDX1 [60]. Similarly, although IL-7 is an important cytokine for B cell development, and IL-4 is a significant B cell growth and differentiation factor, development and numbers of B cells in SCIDX1 appear to be normal.

These apparent paradoxes may be resolved if the cytokines bind to alternative receptors that do not include the γc-chain. We have found recently that IL-7 can elicit production of IL-6 from normal and SCIDX1 monocytes [Clark et al., unpubl. observations]. Although this finding conflicts with the known functional dependence of the IL-7R on the γc-chain [33, 36, 37], it may be explained by IL-7 acting through an alternative receptor that does not include the γc-chain. A low-affinity IL-7 receptor has been identified but not cloned or fully characterised [61]. In addition, a novel IL-7-like cytokine called thymic stromal cell-derived lymphopoietin binds to a receptor which includes the IL-7Rα chain but may not include the γc-chain [62]. It is possible that IL-7 acts on B cell precursors through this second receptor. A second functional IL-7R that also binds thymic stromal cell-derived lymphopoietin would explain why B cell defects are more severe in IL-7R-deficient than γc-chain-deficient mice [62].

The role of the γc-chain in B cell responses to IL-2, IL-4, IL-13 and IL-15 has also been investigated. In these experiments, B cells from 2 SCIDX1 patients with defined mutations in the γc-chain gene and no detectable γc-chain expression were unable to respond to IL-2 or IL-15 confirming the functional importance of the γc-chain in the IL-2R and IL-15R. In contrast, SCIDX1 B cells responded normally to IL-4 and as well or better than control B cells to IL-13 in assays for B cell activation, proliferation, and IgE secretion [63]. These experiments showed either that the γc-chain is not required for signal transduction by IL-4 or IL-13 or that IL-4 and IL-13 can act through an alternative receptor which does not have the γc-chain as a component.

Together, these observations suggest that the phenotype in SCIDX1 and in γc-chain-deficient mice may be ameliorated to some extent by alternative receptors for IL-4 and IL-7 and possibly the IL-9R that do not use the γc-chain.

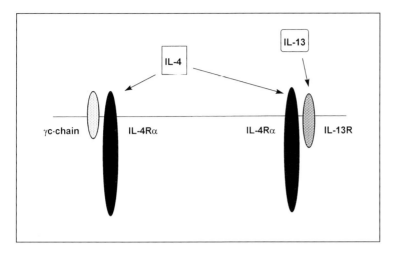

Fig. 1. Model for IL-4R and IL-13R. The IL-4Rα chain is a shared component between the two receptors. IL-4 can bind to both receptors, but IL-13 binds only to the IL-13R.

The IL-13R Does Not Include the γc-Chain and Is a Second Receptor for IL-4

The relationship between the receptors for IL-4 and IL-13 and the functional role of the γc-chain has been examined in more detail in experiments with IL-4 mutant proteins. Functional analysis of IL-4 mutant proteins has identified two sites on the IL-4 protein (site I and site II) important for receptor binding and biological activity, respectively. Site II mutants such as IL-4$_{Y124D}$ bind with almost normal affinity to the IL-4Rα chain but are unable to signal. Recent biochemical experiments and computer modelling of receptor binding have shown that Tyr124 on IL-4 is required for interaction with the γc-chain consistent with an important role for this residue in signal transduction [49, 64]. The IL-4$_{Y124D}$ mutant has been shown to inhibit responses to IL-4 and IL-13 by B cells [65] and the TF1 erythroleukaemic cell line [66] consistent with antagonistic binding to the IL-4Rα chain. IL-4$_{Y124D}$ also inhibits SCIDX1 B cell responses to IL-4 and IL-13 suggesting that both IL-4 and IL-13 can signal through a receptor utilising the IL-4Rα chain but not the γc-chain [41]. Confirmation that the IL-4Rα chain is a component of the IL-13R has been obtained by showing that B cell responses to IL-4 and IL-13 are inhibited by monoclonal antibodies specific for the IL-4Rα chain [39, 67].

These experiments suggest that the IL-4Rα chain is a common component of the receptors or IL-4 and IL-13 (fig. 1). A similar conclusion has been reached recently by Zurawski et al. [69] and Lin et al. [39] and has been confirmed by the recent finding that the cloned mouse and human IL-13 binding proteins associate with the IL-4Rα chain to form receptors for both IL-4 and IL-13 [45, 46].

This model for the IL-4R and IL-13R (fig. 1) has several important functional implications. The most significant of these is that IL-4 can bind to and activate B cells through two different receptors. One of these is the high-affinity IL-4Rα/γc-chain (type I) receptor and the other is the IL-13R complex made up of the IL-4Rα and the IL-13 binding chain (the type II IL-4R). The existence of more than one class of IL-4R has been suggested by earlier binding studies showing high- and low-affinity IL-4 binding sites on human lymphoid cells [69]. Furthermore, functional experiments have shown that 50-fold higher concentrations of IL-4 are required for increased expression of surface CD23 than surface IgM on human B cells consistent with differential binding and activation of high- and low-affinity receptors [70]. Two signalling pathways activated by IL-4 have also been described [71]. High concentrations of IL-4 activate a unique signal transduction pathway in human B cells characterised by rapid and transitory hydrolysis of phosphatidylinositol bisphosphate and calcium mobilisation followed after a short lag period by an increase in cytoplasmic cAMP [71]. IL-13 activation of human monocytes also triggers this signalling pathway [72], and we have found that IL-13 stimulates IP_3 production and increased intracellular cAMP in B cells. On the other hand, IL-4 binding to the high-affinity receptor (IL-4Rα/γc-chain) activates protein tyrosine kinases including Jak1 and Jak3 and phosphorylation of 4PS (IRS-2) [42, 73–76]. Jak1 forms complexes with the IL-4Rα chain [75] and the 4PS protein [75] which has recently been cloned and identified as IRS-2 [74], whereas Jak3 is associated with the γc-chain [27, 29, 76]. The fact that IL-13 activates Jak1 kinase but not Jak3 [42] and that both IL-4 and IL-13 induce phosphorylation of IL-4Rα [77] and activation of STAT6 [40, 42] also implicates the IL-4Rα chain but not the γc-chain as a component of the IL-13R. This model for the IL-13R explains the many overlapping biological properties of IL-4 and IL-13. It also has major implications for the immunodeficiency in SCIDX1 and in construction of receptor antagonists to control IL-4- and IL-13-mediated responses such as IgE production in asthma and allergy.

X-Linked Hyper-IgM Syndrome

The second example of how identifying the gene defect in a primary immunodeficiency has greatly helped our understanding of basic mechanisms in the immune system is HIGM1. Boys with this immunodeficiency have low or absent serum IgG, IgA and IgE but normal or often increased levels of IgM. T cell and B cell numbers are approximately normal. A functional T cell abnormality in these patients was indicated by experiments showing that HIGM1 B cells could be induced to make IgG, IgA and IgE if stimulated with a malignant human T cell clone [78], and more recently by ligation of CD40 and addition of IL-10 or IL-4 [79, 80]. HIGM1 patients are also susceptible to opportunistic infection with *P. carinii* and *Cryptosporidium* more typical of T cell than antibody immunodeficiencies.

CD40L and HIGM1

HIGM1 has been shown to be due to mutations in the T cell activation antigen CD40 ligand (CD40L). CD40L is a type-II integral membrane glycoprotein with significant sequence homology to TNF and a predicted tertiary structure similar to the TNF trimer [81]. It is expressed on activated T cells, mast cells and basophils [82]. In vitro activation of T cells with PMA and a calcium ionophore gives detectable CD40L expression after 1–2 h and optimal expression by 8–10 h. After 24 h expression is rapidly lost. The natural activation signal for CD40L expression in vivo is not known, but it is likely to be TCR ligation plus a second signal important for T cell activation such as B7 binding to CD28. CD40L is expressed strongly on CD4+ and to a much lesser extent on CD8+ T cells with approximately equal distribution between CD45RA and CD45R0 subsets.

CD40L mutations in HIGM1 include deletions giving rise to frame shifts and premature stop codons, or point mutations resulting in single amino acid substitutions [83]. Most identified mutations cluster in the (extracellular) TNF homology domain. One mutation has been found giving a Met_{36}->Arg substitution in the transmembrane signal/anchor domain. The effect of these mutations on CD40L expression by activated T cells was examined by staining PMA/ionomycin-activated T cells from HIGM1 patients with a CD40 human IgFc fusion protein (CD40Fc), a monoclonal CD40L antibody, and a polyclonal antibody (anti-TRAP) raised against a CD40L fusion protein [80]. No staining with CD40 human IgFc fusion protein or CD40 monoclonal antibody was found on activated T cells from any of the HIGM1 patients studied, but normal staining with anti-TRAP was observed in some cases (about half). These findings indicate the presence of mutated CD40L on activated T cells from some patients but the complete loss of the CD40 binding site.

CD40L binding to CD40 is an essential component of T cell interactions with B cells, monocytes, dendritic cells, endothelial cells and probably many other CD40-bearing cells. The importance of this interaction is clear from the devastating effect on immune function mutations in the CD40L gene are known to have in HIGM1 patients, and in murine CD40L and CD40 gene inactivation models [84, 85]. In ecological terms, CD40 may be thought of as a 'keystone' molecule on which many immune functions depend (table 3).

Table 3. Characteristics of HIGM1

Low or absent IgG, IgA and IgE
Normal or elevated levels of IgM
Normal numbers of recirculating B cells
Susceptibility to bacterial and opportunistic infections
    including *P. carinii* and *Cryptosporidium*
No germinal centres
Autoimmunity
Neutropenia
X-linked and autosomal forms
CD40L gene defect in X-linked form

CD40: A Mediator of Intercellular Interactions

CD40 is a type-1 integral membrane glycoprotein belonging to the nerve growth factor receptor superfamily [86]. It is expressed widely on different cell types including B cells, interdigitating cells in T cell zones of secondary lymphoid organs, follicular dendritic cells, thymic epithelia, monocytes, endothelial cells, and some carcinomas [82]. Binding of CD40L expressed on activated T cells to CD40 on each of these cell types results in increased expression of surface activation antigens and secretion of cytokines that are major players in the inflammatory and/or immune response. Antibody or CD40L ligation of CD40 on monocytes or dendritic cells for example increases expression of B7.1 and B7.2 that bind to CD28 or CTLA-4 on T cells as part of the process of antigen presentation. It also stimulates the secretion of cytokines (IL-12, TNFα, IL-1, IFNγ), and activates monocytes to produce NO for killing of micro-organisms [87].

CD40-CD40L-Mediated T-B Cell Interactions

CD40-CD40L interactions are critical for collaboration between T cells and B cells in antibody responses to thymus-dependent antigens. Cross-linking of CD40 on B cells stimulates B cell proliferation which may be enhanced further with anti-IgM or IL-2 or IL-4 [88]. Costimulation with CD40 antibody (or CD40L) and IL-2 or IL-10 stimulates B cells to secrete IgM, IgG and IgA or with IL-4 to give IgE [88, 89]. CD40 ligation has also been shown to rescue CD38+ germinal centre cells from apoptosis [90, 91]. In addition, CD40 apparently gives a signal required for activation of naive B cells to enter the germinal centre and become centrocytes [92] and, on costimulation with IL-2 and IL-10, for the generation of memory B cells in preference to antibody-secreting plasma cells [93, 94]. The importance of these interactions for T cell interactions with B cells in specific antibody responses to thymus-dependent antigens is evident for the absence of

Callard/Smith/Matthews

124

IgG, IgA and IgE antibody in patients with HIGM1 [83]. Similarly, CD40L–/– or CD40–/– mice are unable to respond to TD antigens [84, 85] and normal memory responses are blocked by in vivo blockade of CD40-CD40L interactions [95].

Why Do CD40L Mutations Disrupt High-Affinity IgG, IgA and IgE Antibody Production?

HIGM1 patients do not make significant amounts of IgG, IgA and IgE antibody showing that CD40L expression is essential for normal antibody responses to thymus-dependent antigens. Gene inactivation models or in vivo blockade of other molecules that mediate T cell interactions with B cells do not have such a devastating effect. Why is it then that CD40L-CD40 interactions are so important? One explanation is that CD40 appears to be critical for several B cell functions at different stages of the maturation pathway leading to high-affinity switched antibody-secreting cells (see above). This naturally raises the question: Is it the combined failure of all these CD40-dependent responses that results in the inability to make IgG, IgA or IgE in HIGM1, or is it only one of these functions that is absolutely required? This question is not easy to answer, but it is of major importance for trying to understand why some immunoregulatory molecules such as IL-2 are not essential for normal immune function [57, 96], whereas others like CD40L are absolutely required.

A partial answer to this question for CD40L has been obtained in a recent study of heavy chain switching and affinity maturation in HIGM1 by Razana-jaona et al. [97]. Heavy chain-switched B cells were detected in the blood of 5/5 HIGM1 patients by PCR, although it was not possible to determine what proportion of B cells this represented. In contrast, almost no mutations of the germline VH6 sequence were found consistent with the absence of somatic mutation or affinity maturation in all except 1 HIGM1 patient. These data suggest that some switching may occur in the absence of CD40L expression consistent with reports that other cell surface molecules (such as CD58) may also provide the second signal required for switching [98]. In contrast, normal CD40L expression appears to be essential for B cell somatic mutation and/or rescue from apoptosis. Interestingly, B cells from 1 HIGM1 patient with a mutation in the transmembrane domain that allowed transitory expression of CD40L on T cells after activation had apparently normal levels of somatic mutation [97]. This result shows that partial expression may be all that is required for rescue of B cells from apoptosis in the germinal centre after somatic mutation and escape into the periphery. This particular patient is clinically quite well and is now >30 years old suggesting that partial expression of CD40L may result in a less severe form of the disease. Other male relatives with the same mutation have died from severe infection in infancy however showing that it is not easy to make these sorts of inferences.

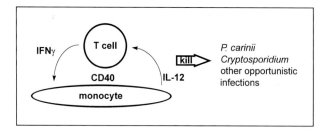

Fig. 2. T cell-monocyte interactions mediated by CD40 generate type I immunity important for killing of *P. carinii* and *Cryptosporidium*.

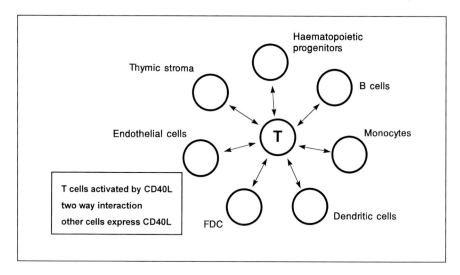

Fig. 3. T cell interactions with many cell types mediated by CD40L-CD40 binding. The interaction in most cases is two-way and can lead to T cell activation as well. FDC = Follicular dendritic cells.

Multiple Roles for CD40

In addition to the inability to make IgG, IgA and IgE, HIGM1 patients are also susceptible to opportunistic infections such as *P. carinii* that are typical of defective cell-mediated immunity. Similarly, mice in which the CD40L or the CD40 gene has been inactivated are susceptible to infection with *Leishmania* [87, 99] and *Pneumocystis* [87]. This has led to a search for CD40 functions in T cell-mediated immunity. Ligation of CD40 activates monocytes to produce NO for microbial killing and pro-inflammatory cytokines including IL-12 that promotes TH1 T cell differentiation [100–102] (fig. 2). IL-12 production by monocytes is impaired in mice with the CD40L gene inactivated. Our own preliminary work has shown that ligation of CD40L on activated T cells promotes IFNγ production in response to PMA and ionomycin. Moreover, T cells from HIGM1 patients activated with PMA and ionomycin made little or no IFNγ or IL-2 consistent with a loss of type-1 (TH1) immunity in the absence of functional CD40L.

CD40 is expressed on many cells other than B cells including dendritic cells and endothelial cells both of which are key players in inflammation and immunity (fig. 3). The expression of CD40 on various cell types is consistent with a wide role for CD40-mediated interactions with activated T cells (and possibly mast cells). It is also important to realise that the various CD40 functions should not be considered in isolation. For example, cytokine production by monocytes activated by CD40 will influence the local inflammatory response and T cell activation and differentiation. In turn, T cells will produce other molecules that will have an impact on monocytes, endothelial cells and B cells. In this way, the immune system is seen to consist of many interacting components which are linked together by (amongst others) CD40-CD40L interactions. In this respect, CD40 can be thought of as a 'keystone' molecule upon which so many different aspects of inflammation and immunity depend.

References

1   Fischer A: Severe combined immunodeficiencies. Immunodefic Rev 1992;3:83–100.
2   Conley ME: Molecular approaches to analysis of X-linked immunodeficiencies. Annu Rev Immunol 1992;10:215–238.
3   Conley ME, Lavoie A, Briggs C, Brown P, Guerra C, Puck JM: Nonrandom X chromosome inactivation in B cells from carriers of X chromosome-linked severe combined immunodeficiency. Proc Natl Acad Sci USA 1988;85:3090–3094.
4   Goodship J, Malcolm S, Lau YL, Pembrey ME, Levinsky RJ: Use of X-chromosome inactivation analysis to establish carrier status for X-linked severe combined immunodeficiency. Lancet 1988;i: 729–732.
5   de Saint Basile G, Arveiler B, Oberle I, Malcolm S, Levinsky RJ, Lau YL, Hofker M, Debre M, Fischer A, Griscelli C, et al: Close linkage of the locus for X-linked severe combined immunodeficiency to polymorphic DNA markers in Xq11–q13. Proc Natl Acad Sci USA 1987;84:7576–7579.
6   Puck JM, Conley ME, Bailey LC: Refinement of linkage of human severe combined immunodeficiency (SCIDX1) to polymorphic markers in Xq13. Am J Hum Genet 1993;53:176–184.
7   Markiewicz S, DiSanto JP, Chelly J, Fairweather N, Le Marec B, Griscelli C, Graeber MB, Muller U, Fischer A, Monaco AP, et al: Fine mapping of the human SCIDX1 locus at Xq12–13.1. Hum Mol Genet 1993;2:651–654.
8   Noguchi M, Yi H, Rosenblatt HM, Filipovich AH, Adelstein S, Modi WS, McBride OW, Leonard WJ: Interleukin-2 receptor gamma chain mutation results in X-linked severe combined immunodeficiency in humans. Cell 1993;73:147–157.
9   Puck JM, Deschenes SM, Porter JC, Dutra AS, Brown CJ, Willard HF, Henthorn PS: The interleukin 2 receptor gamma chain maps to Xq13.1 and is mutated in X-linked severe combined immunodeficiency, SCIDX1. Hum Mol Genet 1993;2:1099–1104.

10   Voss SD, Hong R, Sondel PM: Severe combined immunodeficiency, interleukin 2 (IL-2) and the IL-2 receptor: Experiments of nature continue to point the way. Blood 1994;83:626–635.

11   Nakamura M, Asao H, Takeshita T, Sugamura K: The interleukin 2 receptor heterotrimer complex and intracellular signalling. Semin Immunol 1993;5:309–317.

12   Minami Y, Kono T, Miyazaki T, Taniguchi T: The IL-2 receptor complex: Its structure, function and target genes. Annu Rev Immunol 1993;11:245–267.

13   Giri JG, Kumaki S, Ahdieh M, Friend DJ, Loomis A, Shanebeck K, DuBose R, Cosman D, Park LS, Anderson DM: Identification and cloning of a novel IL-15 binding protein that is structurally related to the alpha chain of the IL-2 receptor. EMBO J 1995;14:3654–3663.

14   Horak ID, Gress RE, Lucas PJ, Horak EM, Waldmann TA, Bolen JB: T lymphocyte interleukin 2 dependent tyrosine protein kinase signal transduction involves the activation of p56lck. Proc Natl Acad Sci USA 1991;88:1996–2000.

15   Torigoe T, Saragovi HU, Reed JC: Interleukin 2 regulates the activity of the lyn protein tyrosine kinase in a B cell line. Proc Natl Acad Sci USA 1992;89:2674–2678.

16   Turner B, Rapp U, App H, Greene M, Dobashi K, Reed J: Interleukin 2 induces tyrosine phosphorylation and activation of p72–74 Raf-1 kinase in a T cell line. Proc Natl Acad Sci USA 1991;88:1227–1231.

17   Evans SW, Farrar WL: Interleukin 2 and diacylglycerol stimulate phosphorylation of 40S ribosomal S6 protein. Correlation with increased protein synthesis and S6 kinase activation. J Biol Chem 1987;262:4624–4630.

18   Asao H, Takeshita T, Nakamura M, Nagata K, Sugamura K: Interleukin 2 (IL-2)-induced tyrosine phosphorylation of IL-2 receptor p75. J Exp Med 1990;171:637–644.

19   Asao H, Kumaki S, Takeshita T, Nakamura M, Sugamura K: IL-2 dependent in vivo and in vitro tyrosine phosphorylation of IL-2 receptor gamma chain. FEBS Lett 1992;304:141–145.

20   Reed JC, Sabath DE, Hoover RG, Prystowsky MB: Recombinant interleukin 2 regulates levels of c-myc mRNA in a cloned murine T lymphocyte. Mol Cell Biol 1985;5:3361–3368.

21   Stern JB, Smith KA: Interleukin 2 induction of T cell G1 progression and c-myb expression. Science 1986;233:203–206.

22   Farrar WL, Cleveland JL, Beckner SK, Bonvini E, Evans SW: Biochemical and molecular events associated with interleukin 2 regulation of lymphocyte proliferation. Immunol Rev 1986;92:49–65.

23   Shibuya H, Yoneyama M, Ninomiya-Tsuji J, Matsumoto K, Taniguchi T: IL-2 and EGF receptors stimulate the haematopoietic cell cylce via different signalling pathways: Demonstration of a novel role for c-myc. Cell 1992;70:57–67.

24   Ihle JN, Kerr IM: Jaks and Stats in signalling by the cytokine receptor superfamily. Trends Genet 1995;11:69–74.

25   Johnston JA, Bacon CM, Finbloom DS, Rees RC, Kaplan D, Shibuya K, Ortaldo JR, Gupta S, Chen YQ, Giri JG, et al: Tyrosine phosphorylation and activation of STAT5, STAT3 and Janus kinases by interleukins 2 and 15. Proc Natl Acad Sci USA 1995;92:8705–8709.

26   Asao H, Takeshita T, Ishii N, Kumaki S, Nakamura M, Sugamura K: Reconstitution of functional interleukin 2 receptor complexes on fibroblastoid cells: Involvement of the cytoplasmic domain of the gamma chain in two distinct signalling pathways. Proc Natl Acad Sci USA 1993;90:4127–4131.

27   Miyazaki T, Kawahara A, Fuji H, Nakagawa Y, Minami Y, Liu Z-J, Oishi I, Silvennoinen O, Witthuhn BA, Ihle JN, et al: Functional activation of Jak1 and Jak3 by selective association with IL-2 receptor subunits. Science 1994;266:1045–1047.

28   Takeshita T, Asao H, Ohtani K, Ishii N, Kumaki S, Tanaka N, Munakata H, Nakamura M, Sugamura K: Cloning of the gamma chain of the human IL-2 receptor. Science 1992;257:379–382.

29   Russell SM, Johnston JA, Noguchi M, Kawamura M, Bacon CM, Friedmann M, Berg M, McVicar DW, Witthuhn BA, Silvennoinen O, et al: Interactions of IL-2 beta and gamma chains with Jak1 and Jak3: Implications for XSCID and XCID. Science 1994;266:1042–1045.

30   Macchi P, Villa A, Giliani S, Sacco MG, Frattini A, Porta F, Ugazio AG, Johnston JA, Candotti F, O'Shea JJ, et al: Mutations of Jak3 gene in patients with autosomal severe combined immunodeficiency (SCID). Nature 1995;377:65–68.

31 Kondo M, Takeshita T, Ishii N, Nakamura M, Watanabe S, Arai K, Sugamura K: Sharing of the interleukin-2 (IL2) receptor gamma chain between receptors for IL-2 and IL-4. Science 1993;262: 1874–1877.

32 Russell SM, Keegan AD, Harada N, Nakamura Y, Noguchi M, Leland P, Friedmann MC, Miyajima A, Puri RK, Paul WF, et al: Interleukin-2 receptor gamma chain: A functional component of the interleukin-4 receptor. Science 1993;262:1880–1883.

33 Kondo M, Takeshita T, Higuchi M, Nakamura M, Sudo T, Nishikawa S-I, Sugamura K: Functional participation of the IL-2 receptor gamma-chain in IL-7 receptor complexes. Science 1994;263: 1453–1454.

34 Kimura Y, Takeshita T, Kondo M, Ishii N, Nakamura M, van Snick J, Sugamura K: Sharing of the IL-2 receptor gamma chain with the functional IL-9 receptor complex. Int Immunol 1995;7:115–120.

35 Giri JG, Ahdieh M, Eisenmann J, Shanebeck K, Grabstein K, Kumaki S, Namen A, Park LS, Cosman D, Anderson D: Utilization of the beta and gamma chains of the IL-2 receptor by the novel cytokine IL-15. EMBO J 1994;143:2822–2830.

36 Noguchi M, Nakamura Y, Russell SM, Ziegler SF, Tsang M, Cao X, Leonard WJ: Interleukin-2 receptor gamma chain: A functional component of the interleukin-7 receptor. Science 1993;262: 1877–1880.

37 Kawahara A, Minami Y, Taniguchi T: Evidence for a critical role for the cytoplasmic region of the interleukin 2 (IL-2) receptor gamma-chain in IL-2, IL-4 and IL-7 signalling. Mol Cell Biol 1994;14: 5433–5440.

38 Yin T, Yang L, Yang Y-C: Tyrosine phosphorylation and activation of Jak family tyrosine kinases by interleukin 9 in MO7E cells. Blood 1995;85:3101–3106.

39 Lin J-X, Migone T-S, Tsang M, Friedmann M, Weatherbee JA, Zhou L, Yamauchi A, Bloom ET, Mietz J, John S, et al: The role of the shared receptor motifs and common Stat proteins in the generation of cytokine pleiotropy and redundancy by IL-2, IL-4, IL-7, IL-13 and IL-15. Immunity 1995;2:331–339.

40 Hou J, Schindler U, Henzel WJ, Ho TC, Brasseur M, McKnight SL: An interleukin 4 induced transcription factor: IL-4 stat. Science 1994;265:1701–1706.

41 Callard RE, Matthews DJ, Hibbert LM: IL-4 and IL-13 receptors: Are they one and the same? Immunol Today 1996;17:108–110.

42 Welham M, Learmonth L, Bone H, Schrader JW: Interleukin 13 signal transduction in lympho-haematopoietic cells. J Biol Chem 1995;270:12286–12296.

43 Obiri NI, Debinski W, Leonard WJ, Puri RK: Receptor for interleukin 13: Interaction with interleukin 4 by a mechanism that does not involve the common gamma chain shared by receptors for interleukins 2, 4, 7, 9 and 15. J Biol Chem 1995;270:8797–8804.

44 Vita N, Lefort S, Laurent P, Caput D, Ferrara P: Characterisation and comparison of the interleukin 13 receptor with the interleukin 4 receptor on several cell types. J Biol Chem 1995;270:3512–3517.

45 Hilton DJ, Zhang J-G, Metcalf D, Alexander WS, Nicola NA, Willson TA: Cloning and characterisation of a binding subunit of the interleukin 13 receptor that is also a component of the interleukin 4 receptor. Proc Natl Acad Sci USA 1996;93:497–501.

46 Caput D, Laurent P, Kaghad M, Lelias JM, Lefort S, Vita N, Ferrara P: Cloning and characterisation of a specific interleukin (IL)-13 binding protein structurally related to the IL-5 receptor alpha chain. J Biol Chem 1996;271:16921–16926.

47 DiSanto JP, Dautry-Varsat A, Certain S, Fischer A, de Saint Basile G: Interleukin-2 (IL-2) receptor gamma chain mutations in X-linked severe combined immunodeficiency disease result in the loss of high affinity IL-2 receptor binding. Eur J Immunol 1994;24:475–479.

48 Ishii N, Asao H, Kimura Y, Takeshita T, Nakamura M, Tsuchiya S, Konno T, Maeda M, Uchiyama T, Sugamura K: Impairment of ligand binding and growth signalling of mutant IL-2 receptor gamma-chains in patients with X-linked severe combined immunodeficiency. J Immunol 1994;153: 1310–1317.

49 Bamborough P, Hedgecock CJR, Richard WG: The interleukin-2 and interleukin-4 receptors studied by molecular modelling. Structure 1994;2:839–851.

50   DiSanto JP, Le Deist F, Caniglia M, Markiewicz S, Lebranchu Y, Griscelli C, Fischer A, de Saint Basile G: Variant forms of X-linked severe combined immunodeficiency disease: One or many genes. Immunodeficiency 1993;4:253–258.
51   Brooks EG, Schmalstieg FC, Wirt DP, Rosenblatt HM, Adkins LT, Lookingbill DP, Rudloff HE, Rakusan TA, Goldman AS: A novel X-linked combined immunodeficiency disease. J Clin Invest 1990;86:1623–1631.
52   Schmalstieg FC, Leonard WJ, Noguchi M, Berg M, Rudloff HE, Denney RM, Dave SK, Brooks EG, Goldman AS: Missense mutation in exon 7 of the common gamma chain gene causes a moderate form of X-linked combined immunodeficiency. J Clin Invest 1995;95:1169–1173.
53   He Y-W, Adkins B, Furse RK, Malek TR: Expression and function of the common gamma chain subunit of the IL-2, IL-4 and IL-7 receptors. J Immunol 1995;154:1596–1605.
54   DiSanto JP, Rieux-Laucat F, Dautry-Varsat A, Fischer A, de Saint Basile G: Defective human interleukin 2 receptor gamma chain in an atypical X chromosome linked severe combined immunodeficiency with peripheral T cells. Proc Natl Acad Sci USA 1994;91:9466–9470.
55   de Saint Basile G, Le Deist F, Caniglia M, Lebranchu Y, Griscelli C, Fischer A: Genetic study of a new X-linked recessive immunodeficiency syndrome. J Clin Invest 1992;89:861–866.
56   DiSanto JP, Keever CA, Small TN, Nichols GL, O'Reilly RJ, Flomenberg N: Absence of interleukin 2 production in a severe combined immunodeficiency disease syndrome with T cells. J Exp Med 1990;171:1697–1704.
57   Schorle H, Holtschke T, Hunig T, Schimpl A, Horak I: Development and function of T cells in mice rendered interleukin-2 deficient by gene targeting. Nature 1991;352:621–624.
58   Kuhn R, Rajewsky K, Muller W: Generation and analysis of interleukin 4 deficient mice. Science 1991;254:707–710.
59   Sadlack B, Kuhn R, Schorle H, Rajewsky K, Muller W, Horak I: Development and proliferation of lymphocytes in mice deficient in both interleukins 2 and 4. Eur J Immunol 1994;24:281–284.
60   Mehler MF, Rozental R, Dougherty M, Spray DC, Kessler JA: Cytokine regulation of neuronal differentiation of hippocampal progenitor cells. Nature 1993;362:62–65.
61   Armitage RJ, Ziegler SF, Friend DJ, Park LS, Fanslow WC: Identification of a novel low-affinity receptor for human interleukin 7. Blood 1992;79:1738–1745.
62   Peschon JJ, Morrissey PJ, Grabstein KH, Ramsdell FJ, Maraskovsky E, Gliniak BC, Park LS, Ziegler SF, Williams DE, Ware CB, et al: Early lymphocyte expansion is severely impaired in interleukin 7 receptor deficient mice. J Exp Med 1994;180:1955–1960.
63   Matthews DJ, Clark PA, Herbert J, Morgan G, Armitage RJ, Kinnon C, Minty A, Grabstein KH, Caput D, Ferrara P, et al: Function of the IL-2 receptor gamma chain in biological responses of X-SCID B cells to IL-2, IL-4, IL-13 and IL-15. Blood 1995;85:38–42.
64   Duschl A: An antagonistic mutant of interleukin 4 fails to recruit the common gamma chain into the receptor complex. Eur J Biochem 1995;228:305–310.
65   Aversa G, Punnonen J, Cocks BG, de Waal Malefyt R, Vega F, Zurawski SM, Zurawski G, De Vries JE: An interleukin 4 (IL-4) mutant protein inhibits both IL-4 or IL-13 induced human immunoglobulin G4 (IgG4) and IgE synthesis and B cell proliferation: Support for a common component shared by IL-4 and IL-13 receptors. J Exp Med 1993;178:2213–2218.
66   Zurawski SM, Vega F, Huyghe B, Zurawski G: Receptors for interleukin 13 and interleukin 4 are complex and share a novel component that functions in signal transduction. EMBO J 1993;12:2663–2670.
67   Renard N, Duvert V, Banchereau J, Saeland S: Interleukin-13 inhibits the proliferation of normal and leukaemic human B cell precursors. Blood 1994;84:2253–2260.
68   Zurawski SM, Chomarat P, Djossou O, Bidaud C, McKenzie ANJ, Miossec P, Banchereau J, Zurawski G: The primary binding subunit of the human interleukin 4 receptor is also a component of the interleukin 13 receptor. J Biol Chem 1995;270:13869–13878.
69   Foxwell BMJ, Woerly G, Ryffel B: Identification of interleukin 4 receptor-associated proteins and expression of both high and low affinity binding on human lymphoid cells. Eur J Immunol 1989;19:1637–1641.
70   Shields JG, Armitage RJ, Jamieson BN, Beverley PCL, Callard RE: Increased expression of surface IgM but not IgD or IgG on human B cells in response to interleukin 4. Immunology 1989;66:224–227.

71 Rigley KP, Thurstan SM, Callard RE: Independent regulation of interleukin 4 (IL-4) induced expression of human B cell surface CD23 and IgM: Functional evidence for two IL-4 receptors. Int Immunol 1991;3:197–203.

72 Sozzani P, Cambon C, Vita N, Seguelas M-H, Caput D, Ferrara P, Pipy B: Interleukin 13 inhibits protein kinase C triggered respiratory burst in human monocytes: Role of calcium and cyclic AMP. J Biol Chem 1995;270:5084–5088.

73 Wang L, Keegan AD, Li W, Lienhard GE, Pacini S, Gutkind JS, Myers MG, Sun X, White MF, Aaronson SA, et al: Common elements in interleukin 4 and insulin signalling pathways in factor dependent haematopoietic cells. Proc Natl Acad Sci USA 1993;90:4032–4036.

74 Sun XJ, Wang L-M, Zhang Y, Yenush L, Meyers MG, Glasheen E, Lane WS, Pierce JH, White MF: Role of IRS-2 in insulin and cytokine signalling. Nature 1995;377:173–177.

75 Yin T, Tsang ML, Yang YC: JAK1 kinase forms complex with interleukin 4 receptor and 4PS/insulin receptor substrate 1 like protein and is activated by interleukin 4 and interleukin 9 in T lymphocytes. J Biol Chem 1994;269:26614–26617.

76 Musso T, Johnston JA, Linnekin D, Varesio L, Rowe TK, O'Shea JJ, McVicar DW: Regulation of JAK3 expression in human monocytes: Phosphorylation in response to interleukins 2, 4, and 7. J Exp Med 1995;181:1425–1431.

77 Smerz-Bertling C, Duschl A: Both interleukin 4 and interleukin 13 induce tyrosine phosphorylation of the 140kDa subunit of the IL-4 receptor. J Biol Chem 1995;270:966–970.

78 Schwaber J, Molgaard H, Orkin SH, Gould HJ, Rosen FS: Early pre-B cells from normal and X-linked agammaglobulinaemia produce C-mu without an attached V_H region. Nature 1983;304:355–358.

79 Durandy A, Schiff C, Bonnefoy J-Y, Forveille M, Rousset F, Mazzei G, Milili M, Fischer A: Induction by anti-CD40 antibody or soluble CD40 ligand and cytokines of IgG, IgA and IgE production by B cells from patients with X-linked hyper-IgM syndrome. Eur J Immunol 1993;23:2294–2299.

80 Callard RE, Smith SH, Herbert J, Morgan G, Padayachee M, Lederman S, Chess L, Kroczek RA, Fanslow WC, Armitage RJ: CD40 ligand (CD40L) expression and B cell function in agammaglobulinaemia with normal or elevated levels of IgM (HIM): A comparison of X-linked, autosomal recessive and non-X-linked forms of the disease, and obligate carriers. J Immunol 1994;153:3295–3306.

81 Korthauer U, Graf D, Mages HW, Briere F, Padayachee M, Malcolm S, Ugazio AG, Notarangeli LD, Levinsky R, Kroczek RA: Defective expression of T-cell CD40 ligand causes X-linked immunodeficiency with hyper-IgM. Nature 1993;361:539–541.

82 Banchereau J, Bazan JF, Blanchard D, Briere F, Galizzi JP, van Kooten C, Liu Y, Rousset F, Saeland S: The CD40 antigen and its ligand. Annu Rev Immunol 1994;12:881–922.

83 Callard RE, Armitage RA, Fanslow WC, Spriggs MK: CD40 ligand and its role in X-linked hyper-IgM syndrome. Immunol Today 1993;14:559–564.

84 Renshaw BR, Fanslow WC, Armitage RJ, Campbell KA, Liggit D, Wright B, Davison BL, Maliszewski CR: Humoral immune responses in CD40 ligand deficient mice. J Exp Med 1994;180:1889–1900.

85 Castigli E, Alt FW, Davidson L, Bottaro A, Mizoguchi E, Bhan AK, Geha RS: CD40 deficient mice generated by recombination-activating gene-2-deficient blastocyst complementation. Proc Natl Acad Sci USA 1994;91:12135–12139.

86 Mallett S, Barclay AN: A new superfamily of cell surface proteins related to nerve growth factor receptor. Immunol Today 1991;12:220–223.

87 Noelle RJ: CD40 and its ligand in host defence. Immunity 1996;4:415–419.

88 Spriggs MK, Armitage RJ, Strockbine L, Clifford KN, Macduff BM, Sato TA, Maliszewski CR, Fanslow WC: Recombinant human CD40 ligand stimulates B cell proliferation and immunoglobulin E secretion. J Exp Med 1992;176:1543–1550.

89 Armitage RA, Macduff BM, Spriggs MK, Fanslow WC: Human B cell proliferation and Ig secretion induced by recombinant CD40 ligand are modulated by soluble cytokines. J Immunol 1993;150:3671–3680.

90 Liu Y, Joshua DE, Williams GT, Smith CA, Gordon JG, MacLennan ICM: The mechanism of antigen-driven selection in germinal centres. Nature 1989;342:929–931.

91 Liu Y, Johnson GD, Gordon J, MacLennan ICM: Germinal centres in T-cell-dependent antibody responses. Immunol Today 1992;13:17–21.
92 Wheeler K, Gordon J: Co-ligation of surface IgM and CD40 on naive B lymphocytes generates a blast population with an ambiguous extrafollicular/germinal centre phenotype. Int Immunol 1996; 8:815–828.
93 Arpin C, Dechanet J, van Kooten C, Merville P, Grouard G, Briere F, Banchereau J, Liu Y-J: Generation of memory B cells and plasma cells in vitro. Science 1995;268:720–722.
94 Foy TM, Laman JD, Ledbetter JA, Aruffo A, Claassen E, Noelle RJ: gp39-CD40 interactions are essential for germinal centre formation and the development of B cell memory. J Exp Med 1994; 180:157–163.
95 Gray D, Dullforce P, Jainandunsing S: Memory B cell development but not germinal centre formation is impaired by in vivo blockade of CD40-CD40L interaction. J Exp Med 1994;180:141–155.
96 Kundig TM, Schorle H, Bachmann MF, Hengartner H, Zinkernagel RM, Horak I: Immune responses in interleukin-2-deficient mice. Science 1993;262:1059–1061.
97 Razanajaona D, van Kooten C, Lebecque S, Bridon J, Ho S, Smith S, Callard RE, Banchereau J, Briere F: The presence of somatic mutations in immunoglobulin V genes correlates with the expression of a partially functional CD40L in X-linked hyper-IgM syndrome. J Immunol, in press.
98 Diaz-Sanchez D, Chegini S, Zhang K, Saxon A: CD58 (LFA-3) stimulation provides a signal for human isotype switching and IgE production distinct from CD40. J Immunol 1994;153:10-20.
99 Soong L, Xu JC, Grewal IS, Kima P, Sun J, Longley BJ, Ruddle NH, McMahon-Pratt D, Flavell RA: Disruption of CD40-CD40 ligand interactions results in an enhanced susceptibility to *Leishmania amazonensis* infection. Immunity 1996;4:263–273.
100 Kiener PA, Moran-Davis P, Rankin BM, Wahl AF, Aruffo A, Hollenbaugh D: Stimulation of CD40 with purified soluble gp39 induces proinflammatory responses in human monocytes. J Immunol 1995;155:4917–4925.
101 Kato T, Hakamada R, Yamane H, Nariuchi H: Induction of IL-12 p40 messenger RNA expression and IL-12 production of macrophages via CD40-CD40 ligand interaction. J Immunol 1996;156: 3932–3938.
102 Alderson MR, Armitage RJ, Tough TW, Strockbine L, Fanslow WC, Spriggs MK: CD40 expression by human monocytes: Regulation by cytokines and activation of monocytes by the ligand for CD40. J Exp Med 1993;178:669–674.

Professor Robin E. Callard, Immunobiology Unit, Institute of Child Health,
30 Guilford Street, London WC1N 1EH (UK)

Subject Index